PHYSICAL FITNESS
the pathway to healthful living

PHYSICAL FITNESS
the pathway to healthful living

ROBERT V. HOCKEY, B.S., M.S., Ed.D.

Professor, Department of Health,
Physical Education, and Recreation,
Northern Michigan University,
Marquette, Michigan

With **109** illustrations

THIRD EDITION

The C. V. Mosby Company

SAINT LOUIS   1977

THIRD EDITION

Copyright © 1977 by The C. V. Mosby Company

All rights reserved. No part of this book may be reproduced
in any manner without written permission of the publisher.

Previous edition copyrighted 1973

Printed in the United States of America

Distributed in Great Britain by Henry Kimpton, London

The C. V. Mosby Company
11830 Westline Industrial Drive, St. Louis, Missouri 63141

Library of Congress Cataloging in Publication Data

Hockey, Robert V
  Physical fitness.

  Bibliography: p.
  Includes index.
  1. Exercise. 2. Physical fitness.
  3. Cardiovascular system. I. Title.
RA781.H57 1977   613.7   76-47675
ISBN 0-8016-2215-8

CB/CB/B 9 8 7 6 5 4 3 2 1

FOREWORD

Dr. Hockey has addressed his text to the concept that given an understanding and appreciation of the vital role of exercise, the thinking citizen will subscribe to regular exercise as a part of his daily routine.

The author has focused, very properly, on the efficiency of the cardiovascular system as basic to the attainment and maintenance of optimal physical fitness. A strong heart, resiliency in arteries and veins, and a profusion of capillaries throughout all tissues—these are the physiological attributes that are far more important than the bulging muscles that the average citizen of today needs less and less.

The novel approach employed by the author involved student participation in alternate lecture and laboratory sessions throughout the semester. The why and how are presented in the classroom, followed in the next session by activity in the gymnasium related to the topic covered in the preceding lecture. Televised lectures presented to large classes increase the efficiency of this part of the instructional program. The size of the laboratory sections is reduced in order to provide the intimate experiences conducive to effective learning. The comprehensive and pertinent subject matter thereby presented develops progressively that body of knowledge which provides the academic and scientific basis for participating in regular physical activity. It is designed to encourage each student to subscribe to a judiciously self-prescribed program of exercise throughout his lifetime.

The program has been successfully initiated as evidenced by requests from college students for activity periods designed to provide them the opportunity to work out periodically throughout the week, after they have completed the course.

It may be appropriate to risk conjecture at this point in stating that the physical education programs which have developed this type of educational experience for their students will long survive—whether the physical education courses are required or elective. This type of approach may prove equally as desirable in the secondary and elementary schools.

The author is to be commended for the timely and scholarly contributions he has made to a phase of physical education in which academic support has been greatly needed.

Dr. Rico Zenti

Retired Chairman, Department of Health,
Physical Education, and Recreation,
Northern Michigan University

v

PREFACE

Physical education programs in the past have had as one of their major objectives the development of skill in one or more sports. Skills have been taught and students have been given an opportunity to participate in these sports during the required physical education classes. It was assumed that participation in these sports would be sufficient to develop and maintain an adequate level of physical fitness. It was also assumed that sports participation would become part of the daily living pattern of a great majority of these students later in life. The validity of both of these assumptions appears to be questionable. Despite the fact that there has been an increase in the amount of leisure time, the average person does not take the time to engage in a regular activity program. He lacks sufficient motivation to make time available for this. This could be because the health benefits that can be derived from regular participation in a well-designed physical fitness program have not been emphasized. If a person can clearly see advantages that can be derived from such a program, he is more likely to be motivated to participate on a regular basis.

This material is presented in the hope that each individual might evaluate his present level of physical fitness, might consider carefully all the information available, and then make a wise decision with regard to the importance of physical activity in his life. Increased knowledge will not contribute to the development of physical fitness, but once an individual is convinced as to the importance of this, then he may have sufficient motivation and sufficient information as to the procedures that he must follow. By careful evaluation of the material presented, a more systematic and intelligent approach to exercise may be possible.

During the past five years or so, many universities across the country have emphasized this academic content associated with health and physical education. Classes have been organized so that this information could be presented to the students. These classes have been referred to as "Fundamentals of Physical Education," "Basic Movement," "An Academic Approach to Physical Education," and "Foundations of Physical Education." Many of these classes have been organized so that the lecture material is presented one day and an additional one or two days are spent each week in the gymnasium. The material in this book is designed for use in such a class as this.

I am indebted to many people for assistance in the production of this book. I would like to thank Dennis Hickey, Jerry Morrow, Betsy Gross, and Marilyn Peterson for their valuable assistance in the preparation of the manuscript, and Dr. Rico Zenti for writing the Foreword. The photographs were taken by Jim Darnton and Don Pavloski, and the students used in these photographs were Shelley Sherman, Debbie Anderson, Tim Furno, Roger Harriman, Darcy Hazel, and John Shrolec.

The drawings were prepared by Eugene Sinervo. I am also indebted to Georgia Horton, Shirley Ruecker, Carol Laituri, and my wife, Judy, for their efforts in preparing parts of this manuscript.

Robert V. Hockey

CONTENTS

ATTITUDE QUESTIONNAIRE*

Initially, it is important to find out how you feel toward exercise and physical education. Each question should be answered by placing an "X" in the appropriate column. Be *honest* in your answers, but at the same time try to be objective. This is an anonymous questionnaire, and the results will not in any way influence your final grade for this course.

Age _____ Sex _____

Laboratory instructor _____

	Strongly agree	Agree	Undecided	Disagree	Strongly disagree
1. Little learning takes place in physical education.					
2. At the college level, physical education classes contribute little and do not justify the time and money spent on them.					
3. Physical education classes should be offered at the college level, but it should be the student's decision as to whether he takes them or not.					
4. Most information relative to exercise and physical fitness is common knowledge.					
5. Physical education should consist of only those activities that are fun to participate in.					
6. I would take physical education classes only if they were a university requirement.					
7. Physical education should develop in a student an understanding of the importance of exercise to health and fitness.					
8. All required subjects at the college level in all areas should be offered only as electives except for the area that the student is majoring in.					
9. Most adults get all the exercise they need by performing their daily tasks.					
10. The development of an adequate level of physical fitness should be a worthwhile objective for all college students.					

*Adapted from Corbin, C. B., Dowell, L. J., Lindsey, R., and Talson, M.: Concepts in physical education, Dubuque, Iowa, 1970, Wm. C. Brown Company, Publishers, p. 146.

ACTIVITY INVENTORY*

At the start of the semester it is also important to determine in which activities you participate regularly and in which activities you would like to improve your skill level.

Place a check mark in column 1 next to each activity that you have participated in regularly for at least 8 weeks any time during the last 12 months.

Place a check mark in column 2 next to each activity that you would like to learn more about and in which you would like to increase your skill level.

Numbers are included next to each activity so that computer cards may be used for tabulating results where desired. Students will use the number corresponding to each activity and make their responses next to that number on the IBM card.

INDIVIDUAL AND DUAL SPORTS

	Col. 1	Col. 2
1. Archery		
2. Badminton		
3. Bowling		
4. Calisthenics		
5. Fencing		
6. Fly casting		
7. Golf		
8. Gymnastics		
9. Handball		
10. Hiking		
11. Jogging		
12. Judo		
13. Paddle ball		
14. Skating		
15. Skiing		
16. Tennis		
17. Track and field		
18. Weight lifting		
19. Wrestling		

DANCE

	Col. 1	Col. 2
20. Ballet		
21. Ballroom		
22. Creative		
23. Folk		
24. Square		

TEAM SPORTS

	Col. 1	Col. 2
25. Baseball		
26. Basketball		
27. Field hockey		
28. Ice hockey		
29. Softball		
30. Soccer		
31. Touch football		
32. Volleyball		

AQUATICS

	Col. 1	Col. 2
33. Canoeing		
34. Diving		
35. Lifesaving		
36. Sailing		
37. Swimming		
38. Water safety instruction (WSI)		

OTHERS (list)

	Col. 1	Col. 2

*Adapted from Humphrey, J. H., and Ingram, A. G.: Introduction to physical education for college students, Boston, 1969, Holbrook Press, p. 37.

T   F

___ ___ **1.** Physical education activity classes are required in only a small number of universities and colleges.

___ ___ **2.** A physically educated person could be defined as one who is physically fit.

___ ___ **3.** Most college students have the necessary motivation to participate regularly in some form of physical activity.

___ ___ **4.** The main reason why many people are not more active is that they just do not have sufficient time to exercise.

___ ___ **5.** Keeping students occupied and letting them have fun and play games are probably the most important objectives of a good physical education program.

___ ___ **6.** More people now appear to be concerned about exercise and fitness than previously in this country.

___ ___ **7.** Gaining knowledge concerning physical fitness will definitely contribute to an improvement in the level of physical fitness.

___ ___ **8.** The human body has experienced little or no difficulty in adapting to increased mechanism in today's society.

chapter 1
A new approach to physical education

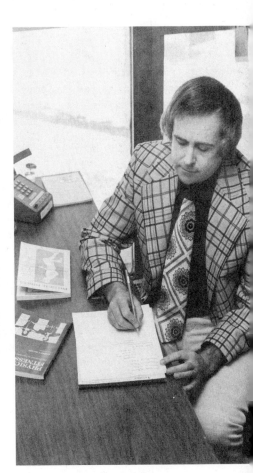

Physical education may be defined simply as that integral part of total education that contributes to the development of the individual through some form of physical activity. It must involve a carefully planned sequence of learning experiences designed to fulfill the growth, development, and behavior needs of each student.

PHYSICAL EDUCATION—A REQUIREMENT OR AN ELECTIVE?

Each day thousands of young men and women take part in some organized physical education program—a requirement at many colleges and universities. A recent survey indicated that 94% of the 723 universities sampled have a physical education requirement.[8] This requirement varies considerably, ranging from one semester to four years. However, the majority of these universities require the students to satisfactorily complete two years of physical education to satisfy the graduation requirement. Fraleigh and Gustafson[4] indicate that in a free and democratic society it is usually accepted that for something to be required exposure to it must be essential to the well-being of those for whom it is required.

Many college students lack an understanding of the potential values of participation in physical education activities and believe that physical education is a waste of time and has little to contribute to their total education. The fact that such a large number of universities and colleges require physical education indicates that there is nearly unanimous agreement that physical education does play an important part in the total education of college students.

As freshmen and sophomores, most students find that there are a large number of subjects that must be taken. Many students resent having to take these courses because most of them appear to have little to do with their major areas of specialization. However, these courses are required in an attempt to expose students to the "general" education considered desirable for American youth. For many of them it is probably difficult to understand why so many universities require physical education. This may be an indication that most high school students in the United States have not been exposed to good physical education programs. Certainly this is a generalization; however, if high schools were doing an adequate job as far as training youth in proper physical education skills and knowledge is concerned, students would not be asking why they have to take physical education. Also, people would be free of a tremendous number of physical and mental disabilities.[9]

Sanborn and Hartman present some interesting information in support of required physical education. Their results are summarized as follows:

1. Studies among students indicate that they prefer physical education to be required.
2. A large majority of colleges require physical education.
3. Regular physical activity is absolutely necessary as one contributing factor to the health and physical fitness necessary for the pursuit of exacting studies.

4. If it is placed on an elective basis, those who need physical education will *not* elect it.
5. Very few college freshmen can be considered to be physically educated.[13]

IMPORTANCE OF THE ACADEMIC APPROACH TO PHYSICAL EDUCATION

The report of the President's Commission on Higher Education states that "college programs of physical education should provide an opportunity for the student to put into practice his theoretical knowledge of healthful habits."[10] This statement implies that there is a theoretical body of knowledge associated with physical education. Unfortunately, students graduating from high school in most cases have not been exposed to this knowledge. Many high school programs are directed entirely toward the development of sports skills or physical fitness, or both. These are important but should not constitute the entire high school program. As a student progresses through high school, he should be brought into contact with the more academic elements of physical education.[16]

At present this situation does not exist, although it appears that its adoption would be received favorably in at least one state in this country. Oseness and Joyce[7] interviewed physical educators, coaches, administrators, and health educators in the state of Kansas with regard to the possible adoption of a new curriculum for high school physical education. The curriculum that was proposed included information relating to the value of physical activity to the human body. It also utilized lecture and laboratory sessions aimed at assisting the student in understanding himself and the benefits that could be derived from physical activity. The results of this study indicate that there is a definite need for such a curriculum change and that the quantity of academic content included in high school physical education programs should be increased. Other positive indications from this study were as follows:

1. It was generally believed that the public would accept such a program.
2. The proposed program had more carry-over potential than the existing program.
3. Only 8% of the eighty high school personnel interviewed indicated that they would *not* be willing to try such a program as this.

Such a change would be difficult to initiate, and much time would be involved in implementing such a program. Although this information is not now being presented at the high school level, many universities across the country have incorporated this body of knowledge into their required physical education programs. This new approach has been classified as an academic approach to physical education.

Wireman indicates that physical education has achieved only low educational status and a low degree of academic respectability because it has emphasized the physical rather than the academic aspects and that physical education has been "too far removed from the main educational stream."[16]

The following objectives are presented in an attempt to identify the information associated with physical education that appears to be important. Each student should (1) acquire knowledge of the structure and functioning of the human body; (2) understand fully the role of exercise in improving one's level of physical fitness so that each can decide how much is necessary and what kind of activity is best; (3) develop an understanding of the physiological benefits that can be derived from regular exercise; (4) understand the principles involved in conducting a good exercise or training program and be able to develop an acceptable program; (5) attain knowledge concerning the fundamental relationship between exercise, diet, and weight control.

CRITERIA FOR A GOOD PHYSICAL EDUCATION PROGRAM

The American public has been misinformed concerning what constitutes a good physical education program and what values can be attained through regular participation in such a program. Many people still confuse athletics with physical education.

A person who has been exposed to a good physical education program should be able to respond positively to the following questions:

Yes   No

1. Do you understand how your body functions and the changes that take place as a result of regular exercise?

2. Do you understand the effects of various types and intensities of activities on your body?

3. Can you design an activity program to meet your present and future needs?

4. Do you know how to evaluate your present level of physical fitness? Can you?

5. Do you have adequate knowledge and skill in a sufficient number of activities so that you can enjoy participation in these activities throughout all seasons of the year regardless of geographic location or the facilities available?

6. Do you understand the values of regular physical activity and particularly its role in maintaining a healthy, more efficient body?

7. Do you participate regularly in an exercise program designed to develop and maintain an adequate level of physical fitness?

8. Do you maintain an adequate level of physical fitness by having a body capable of meeting the daily demands made upon it without experiencing undue fatigue?

9. Do you demonstrate adequate social adjustment by reacting favorably to such things as winning, losing, adversity, team play, and competition?

10. Do you demonstrate a feeling of self-confidence by being aware of your strengths and weaknesses, your abilities and limitations, and by being concerned about your appearance?

The above examples give some idea of the philosophies behind certain types of programs that are being developed at the college level and the academic content within these programs. It is apparent that being physically educated is indeed an important part of total education. These programs seek to answer some of the typical questions that frequently are presented at the college level—What is the unique purpose of physical education in the college? What does the program have to offer students that is considered important enough to permit it to continue to assume its present status? Should academic credit be given for physical education at the college level? How these questions are answered will depend on how physical education is conceived. Unfortunately, many persons have an entirely false concept of physical education. As Blackenbury indicates, "The day may be gone when the gym teacher unlocks the door, throws out the ball, and turns his attention to such weightier matters as plotting defensive strategy for the football team."[2] This situation, however, still exists in many of our schools. To a large percentage of adults in this country, physical education means nothing more than "fun and games" for the students. Some physical educators believe that keeping the students "occupied" is all that is necessary as far as physical education is concerned. A re-education of many adults, teachers, and students is necessary.

LOW LEVEL OF PHYSICAL FITNESS IN THE UNITED STATES

Today more people in the United States appear to be interested in exercise and fitness. A recent article indicates that 60 million Americans are on a "fitness kick." The information presented in this article indicates that "millions of Americans—in the largest numbers ever—are turning to strenuous physical exercise as an escape from the illness, fatigue, and boredom of today's sedentary way of life."[15]

Behind all of this interest in exercise is a growing awareness of the apparent low level of physical fitness and the apparent deteriorating physical condition of many Americans. The seriousness of this problem can be ascertained after consideration of the following facts:

1. Approximately 55% of all deaths in the United States result from cardio-vascular diseases of the heart and blood vessels. Many of these deaths are directly associated with obesity and inactivity.
2. Over 50% of adults in this country can be considered to be overweight.
3. Low back pain is a serious problem costing industry over $1 billion annually in lost goods and services and approximately $225 million in workmen's compensation.[1] It has been estimated that 80% of low back pain problems are due to improper muscular development and result from lack of regular exercise.
4. The American population pays an estimated $35 million each year for worthless methods aimed at improving physical fitness or losing weight the easy "no work" way.[17]

The situation in this country could well have resulted from the poor physical education programs that have been offered at high school and college levels in the past. President Kennedy presented an excellent summary of the situation in his article "The Soft American," in which he indicated the following:

the harsh fact of the matter is that there is an increasingly large number of young Americans who are neglecting their bodies—whose physical fitness is not what it should be—who are getting soft. Such softness on the part of individual citizens can help to strip and destroy the vitality of a nation.[6]

The reason why more adults do not participate regularly in some form of physical activity is at present uncertain. It could be that the lack of academic content in physical education classes in past years now is reflected in the attitudes of many adults and in the decisions that many of them make. For example, many adults who do not participate in a regular program of physical activity will indicate when asked why that there is just not sufficient time for this. It is rather interesting, however, that these same people usually take time to watch their favorite basketball team, football team, or television program, or to engage in some form of "passive" relaxation. It has been estimated that the average American family watches television 5 hours daily. It is no wonder that the American population has been referred to as a nation of spectators.

Time, obviously, is not the explanation. People can usually find time to do what they want to do. In recent years there has been a tremendous increase in the amount of leisure time available to each individual. This has come about mainly because of decreased time spent at work. This relationship, showing the trend over the last 50 years, is presented in Fig. 1-1. Whether this increased amount of leisure time is good or not depends on its use. If used as many Americans use it today, in aimless play and in various forms of passive amusement, then it is obviously not good for them or for society. One of the

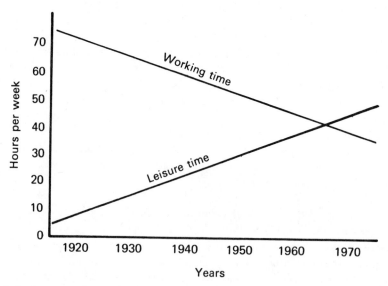

Fig. 1-1. Decrease in work time and increase in leisure—1920 to 1970. (Adapted from Van Huss, Niemeyer, Olson, and Friedrick.[14])

major aims of physical education classes should be to reverse the trend toward physical inactivity and thus to lessen the amount of physical degeneration in our society.

A recent survey[12] indicated that approximately 30% of the subjects who did not exercise listed "not enough time" as the reason they did not exercise. Twenty-five percent indicated that they "get enough exercise by working." Approximately 16% cited "medical reasons" as their excuse while approximately 10% considered that they were too old to exercise.

The President's Council suggests several ways of persuading people to exercise regularly: (1) show them how to fit exercise into their busy schedules; (2) convince older people that age is no barrier to exercise; (3) appeal to their concern for health and an attractive appearance; (4) convince them that exercise can be enjoyable; and (5) present more information to them on the types of exercise that are best and the amount of exercise necessary to develop and maintain adequate fitness.

The President's Council on Physical Fitness further suggests the following:

> No longer can we afford to consider anyone fully educated until he knows how—and is thoroughly motivated—to keep himself in the best possible physical condition at all times. Achieving this end for all students should be one of the primary goals of every college.[11]

The existing situation implies that each member of society must choose how this increased leisure time is to be spent. If the stated objectives of physical education are achieved, it is anticipated that more students will be motivated to participate regularly in physical activity. The student who has been exposed to the academic body of knowledge relating to physical education will be in a position to make a much wiser decision when he has a full understanding of the facts.

It also seems to be important in physical education to teach those activities and to encourage students to take those activities that have some carry-over value—the ones in which adults can participate in later life. Blackenbury states:

> man always finds time to do what he wants to do and people tend to enjoy doing the things they do well. If students learn the basic skills essential to good performance, and if they learn them in an atmosphere they find pleasant, it is likely their learning will become the basis for many hours of enjoyment as adults.[2]

SUMMARY

It appears as though motivation is the key to getting a person to exercise. Just increasing an individual's knowledge concerning exercise and physical fitness is not enough; he must change his attitude toward regular exercise. If he believes strongly enough in physical activity and exercise, he will want to do something about it. For many persons an understanding of the benefits that can be derived from exercise is sufficient motivation for them to engage in some form of regular physical activity. One would hope that as a result of material contained in this book many students will be motivated to devise their own exercise program and make exercise a part of their daily living habits.

REFERENCES

1. Allsen, Phillip E., Harrison, Joyce M., and Vance, Barbara: Fitness for life, Dubuque, Iowa, 1975, William C. Brown Company, Publishers, p. 1.
2. Blackenberry, R. L.: Physical education. An intellectual emphasis? Quest, Dec., 1963, p. 3.
3. Corbin, C. B., Dowell, L. J., and Landis, C. W.: Concepts and experiments in physical education, Dubuque, Iowa, 1968, William C. Brown Company, Publishers, p. 2.
4. Fraleigh, W. P., and Gustafson, W. F.: Can we defend required programs? Journal of Health, Physical Education, and Recreation **35:**32, Feb., 1964.
5. Humphrey, J. H., and Ingram, A. G.: Introduction to physical education for college students, Boston, 1969, Holbrook Press, p. 37.
6. Kennedy, J. F.: The Soft American, Sports Illustrated, Dec. 26, 1960, p. 15.
7. Oseness, W. H., and Joyce, P. J.: An analysis of attitudes toward certain recommended changes in the physical education curriculum. Paper presented at 1969 American Association for Health, Physical Education, and Recreation, Central District Convention, St. Paul, Minn.
8. Oxendine, J. B.: Status of required physical education programs in colleges and universities, Journal of Health, Physical Education, and Recreation **40:**32, Jan., 1969.
9. Penman, K. A.: Physical education for college students, ed. 2, St. Louis, 1968, The C. V. Mosby Co., p. 6.
10. President's Commission on Higher Education: Higher education for American democracy. Establishing the goals, New York, 1948, Harper & Brothers, p. 54.
11. President's Council on Physical Fitness: Fitness and leadership: Suggestions for colleges and universities, Washington, D.C., 1964, U.S. Government Printing Office.
12. President's Council on Physical Fitness and Sports: Newsletter, April, 1976, p. 16.
13. Sanborn, M. A., and Hartman, B.: Issues in physical education, Philadelphia, 1964, Lea & Febiger.
14. Van Huss, W., Niemeyer, R., Olson, H., and Frederick, J.: Physical activity in modern living, ed. 2, Englewood Cliffs, N.J., 1969, Prentice-Hall, Inc., p. 3.
15. Why are 60 million Americans on a fitness kick? U.S. News and World Report, Jan. 14, 1974, pp. 26-28.
16. Wireman, B. O.: What are the underlying values in physical education? The Physical Educator **22:**55, May, 1965.
17. Wyden, P., and Wyden, B.: Why diet and exercise fads don't turn your fatness into fitness. In The healthy life, New York, 1966, Time, Inc.

T   F

___ ___ **1.** The function of the left side of the heart is to circulate purified blood to all parts of the body.

___ ___ **2.** Veins always carry used blood back to the heart.

___ ___ **3.** The size of the heart cannot increase with exercise.

___ ___ **4.** The purpose of the valves in the circulatory system is to regulate the flow of blood by allowing it to flow in only one direction.

___ ___ **5.** People who have desk jobs are more likely to have varicose veins than those who are more active.

___ ___ **6.** A conditioned man may have a resting heart rate that is 20 beats per minute slower than the untrained man.

___ ___ **7.** A reduction in the resting heart rate as a result of training will reduce the amount of oxygen delivered to the muscles.

___ ___ **8.** The force of the heart is largely responsible for the return of blood through the veins to the heart.

___ ___ **9.** A low resting heart rate is a good indication the heart is not functioning efficiently.

___ ___ **10.** The best way to recover following a strenuous task is to lie down immediately.

chapter 2
The cardiovascular system

The word *cardiovascular* refers to the heart and blood vessels, which make up the life stream of the human body. Information relating to the construction and function of the heart and circulatory system is presented so that some of the problems associated with heart disease may be better understood.

THE HEART AS A MUSCULAR PUMP

The heart is simply a muscular pump that provides the force necessary to keep the blood circulating throughout the network of arteries. This hollow, muscular organ is located between the lungs and the diaphragm in what is known as the medial sternal space. It is mostly to the left of the midline of the body with its apex pointing down.

It can actually be considered to consist of two pumps. A thick muscular wall known as the *septum* divides the heart cavity down the middle into what is known as a *right heart* and a *left heart*.

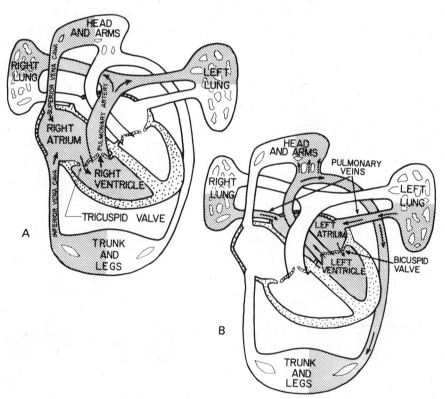

Fig. 2-1. A, Blood flow associated with right heart. Note that major purpose of right heart is to pump blood to lungs, where oxygen is picked up and carbon dioxide eliminated. **B,** Blood flow associated with left heart. Note that left heart is responsible for pumping blood out of left ventricle via the aorta to all parts of body. (Drawings by Eugene Sinervo.)

On each side is an upper chamber known as the atrium and a lower chamber called the ventricle. Each atrium is separated from the ventricle below by a valve, which regulates the flow of blood.[5] These are referred to as atrioventricular valves.

The *right heart* receives blood that has completed its cycle through the body. This blood collects in the right atrium of the heart. Actually this used blood from the body reaches the heart by two large veins—the superior and inferior venae cavae. The superior vena cava returns blood from the head and the arms while the inferior vena cava drains the blood from the trunk and the legs. A third opening into the right atrium is the coronary sinus. This returns blood that is used by the heart muscle itself. From the right atrium the blood enters the right ventricle through the tricuspid valve. The blood is pumped from the right ventricle through the pulmonary arteries to the lungs, where it picks up fresh oxygen and gives up carbon dioxide. The function of the right heart, then, is to pump blood to the lungs, where oxygen is picked up and carbon dioxide is eliminated. The blood flow associated with the right heart is illustrated in Fig. 2-1, *A*.

The *left heart* receives the reoxygenated blood, which is returned through the pulmonary veins.[5] This blood collects in the left atrium and passes from this upper chamber to the lower, through the mitral, or bicuspid, valve. It is this left ventricle that pumps the blood out of the heart. The blood passes through the aorta—the largest artery in the body—to all parts of the body. Fig. 2-1, *B*, illustrates the blood flow associated with the left heart.

VALVES OF THE HEART

The valves play an important role in regulating the flow of blood. Besides the two atrioventricular valves that have been explained previously, two other valves are located where the pulmonary artery and aorta join the ventricles. These valves as well as the two atrioventricular valves are unidirectional and allow blood to flow in only one direction. These prevent the backward flow of blood during diastole, when the heart is relaxed. The heart sounds that may be heard with a stethoscope are caused by the closing of the valves of the heart. The sound that is heard is lubb-dupp. The first of these sounds is caused by the atrioventricular valves as they close when the contraction of the ventricles takes place. At this time the other two valves, the aortic and pulmonary valves, are open as blood is being ejected from the heart. The dupp sound is made by the closing of the valves in the aorta and pulmonary arteries as the heart again is filling with blood.

BLOOD VESSELS

A clear distinction is necessary between arteries and veins. Any vessel taking blood away from the heart is an artery, whereas any vessel returning blood to the heart is a vein. A knowledge of the structure of the artery is most important in understanding heart disease. The cross sections of an artery and vein are compared in Fig. 2-2.[3] Notice that both arteries and veins have three layers:

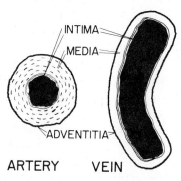

INTIMA
MEDIA
ADVENTITIA
ARTERY   VEIN

Fig. 2-2. Comparison between cross section of an artery and a vein. Note that muscular wall (media) of artery is much thicker than that of vein. (Drawing by Eugene Sinervo.)

(1) intima, or innermost layer, (2) media, or middle layer, and (3) adventitia, or outer layer. However, the muscular wall of the normal artery is much thicker than that of the vein. This allows the arteries to be elastic so that when blood is ejected from the heart they can expand to receive the blood. During the relaxation phase of the cardiac cycle, the muscular walls of the arteries then contract to keep the blood moving through the arterial system.

The arterial branches eventually become smaller and smaller. The smallest branches are known as *capillaries*. It is here that the oxygen and nutrients leave the blood and enter the body cells and that carbon dioxide and metabolic wastes leave the cells and are picked up by the bloodstream.

As fatty deposits accumulate on the inner arterial walls, they tend to lose their elasticity and become smaller in size. This decreases the ability of the circulatory system to function efficiently and increases the possibility of cardio-vascular problems.

Blood is returned to the heart through the network of veins. As indicated, these veins do not have the thick, muscular walls that most arteries have. For this reason there is less pressure in the veins. This does not create a problem for blood returning from the upper parts of the body, since gravity will assist in the return of this blood to the heart.[4] However, blood in the arms and legs must rely on the squeezing action of the muscles in order to be returned to the heart. There is a system of valves in the veins that allows the blood to flow only toward the heart. These veins are located between the skeletal muscles, and when the muscles contract, these veins are "squeezed" and the blood flows toward the heart. If too much time is spent standing at attention, it is not uncommon for a person to experience fatigue and to pass out. Blood is not returned from the lower parts of the body to the heart, and it "pools" in these lower areas. Varicose veins result from the failure of used blood to be returned to the heart at a "fast enough" rate. The accumulated blood causes the veins to swell. Varicose veins occur frequently in individuals whose jobs require that they stand for a number of hours each day or who remain seated for extended periods of time.

BASIC TERMS ASSOCIATED WITH THE CARDIOVASCULAR SYSTEM

Certain basic terms associated with the cardiovascular system need to be explained to understand the material that is presented later. These basic terms include (1) heart rate, (2) stroke volume, (3) cardiac output, and (4) blood pressure.

Heart rate

For an average untrained person in the resting condition, the heart beats approximately seventy-two times per minute. This is known as the heart rate, or pulse. It is caused by the impact of the blood on the arteries as the heart contracts. It can be detected easily by placing a finger on the radial artery located on the lateral side of the wrist or at one of the carotid arteries that pass anteriorly in the neck. In children this rate is much faster, whereas in the highly trained individual the heart becomes more efficient, and the resting heart rate is often much lower.*

Stroke volume

Each time the heart contracts, a certain amount of blood is ejected. This is known as the stroke volume, which is defined as the amount of blood ejected with each beat of the heart. In the resting condition for an untrained person the stroke volume is approximately 70 ml.

Cardiac output

The cardiac output is defined as the amount of blood that the heart is able to circulate each minute. It is dependent on the stroke volume and the heart rate.

$$\text{Cardiac output} = \text{Heart rate} \times \text{Stroke volume}$$

Using the average figures presented previously, the average cardiac output is calculated as follows:

$$
\begin{aligned}
\text{Cardiac output} &= \text{Heart rate} \times \text{Stroke volume} \\
&= 72 \times 70 \\
&= 5{,}040 \text{ ml/min} \\
&= 5.04 \text{ l./min}
\end{aligned}
$$

This means that for a person in the resting condition approximately 5 liters of blood are circulated by the heart each minute.†

Blood pressure

Blood pressure is the amount of force that the blood exerts against the artery walls. It is usually expressed in millimeters of mercury and is the force that keeps the blood flowing through the arteries. It is generated by the heart as it contracts and is maintained by the elasticity of the artery walls. Everyone has blood pressure, for without it the blood would not circulate.[1]

---

*These training effects are discussed in detail in Chapter 10.
†A liter (l.) is approximately equivalent to a quart.

Each time the heart contracts, the blood pressure goes up. The contraction phase of the cardiac cycle is defined as systole; thus this upper blood pressure is referred to as the systolic blood pressure. Each time the heart relaxes, the blood pressure decreases. The relaxation phase of the cardiac cycle is referred to as diastole, and hence the lower blood pressure is known as diastolic blood pressure. Blood pressure is written as systolic/diastolic. For example, 120/80 indicates that the systolic blood pressure is 120 mm of mercury while the diastolic blood pressure is 80 mm.

In measuring blood pressure, the physician uses a sphygmomanometer (Fig. 2-3). An airtight cuff is wrapped around the arm just above the elbow. The cuff is connected to a glass tube filled with mercury. Air is pumped into the cuff by squeezing a bulb. As the cuff becomes tighter, it compresses a large artery in the arm—the brachial artery. This temporarily cuts off the flow of blood to the forearm, and no heart sound can be heard when a stethoscope is placed on the compressed artery just below the cuff. As the air pressure in the cuff is released, the mercury level drops. Eventually a point will be reached at which the blood pressure in the artery is just greater than the air pressure in the cuff. Blood will now begin to flow through the artery, and the heart sound may be heard by using the stethoscope. This is the systolic or upper pressure—it is the maximum pressure that can be produced by the heart.

As the physician continues to let air out of the cuff, the sounds heard through the stethoscope will become louder as more blood passes through the artery. Finally, a point will be reached at which the distinct heart sounds disappear as the blood is flowing steadily through the artery. At this point the

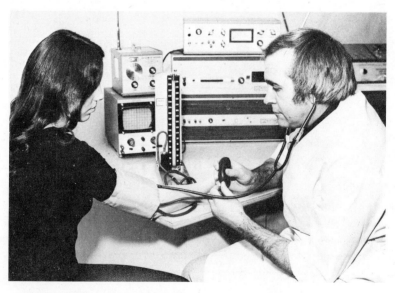

Fig. 2-3. Measurement of blood pressure with sphygmomanometer.

Table 2-1. Normal blood pressure for college-age men and women*

Sex	Blood pressure	Mean	Standard deviation
Male	Systolic	123	13.7
Male	Diastolic	76	9.9
Female	Systolic	116	11.8
Female	Diastolic	72	9.7

*From Lasser, R. P., and Master, A. M.: Mean resting blood pressure in apparently healthy persons 20 to 106 years of age, Geriatrics **14:**345, 1959.

height of the mercury shows the diastolic or lower pressure representing the least amount of pressure in the artery.[1] The average, or normal, blood pressure figures for college-age men and women are presented in Table 2-1.

SUMMARY

The circulatory system is a most important system, for all other systems of the body depend on it. As energy is required for the performance of all activity, the efficiency with which the body can circulate the blood is an important factor in the determination of the amount of work that the body can perform. Also, by having a complete knowledge of the construction and function of the circulatory system it will be possible to understand more fully certain aspects of cardiovascular disease.

REFERENCES

1. High blood pressure, New York, 1966, American Heart Association, p. 3.
2. Prinzmetal, M., and Winter, W.: Heart attack; new hope, new knowledge, new life, New York, 1965, Simon & Schuster, Inc., p. 17.
3. United States Department of Health, Education, and Welfare: The circulatory system, Public Health Service publication no. 482, Washington, D.C., 1964, U.S. Government Printing Office, p. 16.
4. Varicose veins, New York, 1961, American Heart Association, p. 5.
5. The wonderful human machine, Chicago, 1961, American Medical Association, p. 26.

ADDITIONAL READINGS

Corbin, C. B., Dowell, L. J., and Landiss, C. W.: Concepts and experiments in physical education, Dubuque, Iowa, 1968, Wm. C. Brown Company, Publishers.
Miller, B. F., and Burt, J. J.: Good health, personal and community, Philadelphia, 1966, W. B. Saunders Company.
Reduce your risk of heart attack, New York, 1966, American Heart Association, p. 4.
Turner, C. E.: Personal and community health, ed. 14, St. Louis, 1971, The C. V. Mosby Co.
Wyden, P., and Wyden, B.: Why diet and exercise fads won't turn your fatness into fitness. In The healthy life, New York, 1966, Time, Inc., pp. 24-25.

chapter 3
Cardiovascular disease and associated risk factors

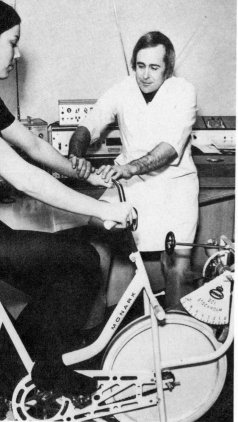

T   F

— — **1.** A person who has smoked for 5 years cannot reduce his chances of a heart attack by discontinuing this habit.

— — **2.** Smoking is related to the incidence of heart disease because it causes an imbalance in the oxygen content of the blood.

— — **3.** Diastolic blood pressure is lower than systolic pressure because it represents the pressure in the arteries during the refilling phase of the cardiac cycle.

— — **4.** Cholesterol is not essential to the normal functioning of the body.

— — **5.** Vigorous exercise is not recommended by physicians for prevention of heart disease.

— — **6.** Females have fewer heart attacks than males.

— — **7.** Postmen have fewer heart attacks than postal clerks.

— — **8.** High blood pressure and obesity are positively related.

— — **9.** Of all the civilized countries the incidence of heart disease in the United States is greater per 100,000 of population than in any other country.

When the functioning of any part of the circulatory system is impaired, blood is not supplied in sufficient quantity to various parts of the body. The areas affected then are deprived of a sufficient supply of oxygen. The heart, like every other organ of the body, is subject to disease. Damage may occur in the heart itself, or it may occur in any of the vessels carrying the blood. Disease of this type is referred to as cardiovascular disease rather than heart disease.

Cardiovascular disease is not a single disease but includes a number of specific diseases. The major cardiovascular diseases are listed in Fig. 3-1, together with the percentage of total cardiovascular deaths attributable to each. These figures indicate that coronary heart disease and stroke together account for 76% of all deaths attributable to cardiovascular disease.[5]

Cardiovascular disease has been the leading cause of death in this country since 1920 and at present accounts for approximately 55% of all deaths.[31] A summary of the major causes of death in the United States is presented in Fig. 3-2.

The death rate attributable to cardiovascular disease has continued to rise sharply in recent years. In 1900, for example, only 20% of all deaths were charged to these causes, whereas in 1963 the corresponding figure was 54.8%.[31]

Table 3-1. Leading causes of death in the United States for 1900 and 1965*

Cause of death 1900	Death rate per 100,000 of population of all ages	Cause of death 1965	Death rate per 100,000 of population of all ages
1. Tuberculosis	194.4	1. Diseases of the heart	367.2
2. Pneumonia	175.4	2. Cancer	153.5
3. Diarrhea and enteritis	139.9	3. Stroke	103.7
4. Diseases of the heart	137.4	4. Accidents	55.7
5. Nephritis	88.7	5. Influenza and pneumonia	31.9
6. Diseases of infancy	72.3	6. Diseases of infancy	28.6
7. Stroke	72.0	7. Arteriosclerosis	19.7
8. Accidents	66.6	8. Diabetes mellitus	17.1
9. Cancer	64.0	9. Cirrhosis of the liver	12.8
10. Bronchitis	45.3	10. Suicide	11.1
11. Meningitis	40.6	11. Congenital malformations	10.1
12. Diphtheria	40.3	12. Emphysema	9.6
13. Typhoid fever	31.3	13. Nephritis	6.2
14. Influenza	26.7	14. Hypertension	6.0
15. Paralysis	26.2	15. Homicide	5.5

*From Diehl, H. S., and Dalrymple, W.: Healthful living, New York, 1968, McGraw-Hill Book Company, p. 10.

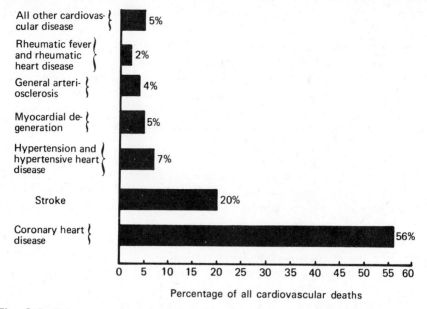

Fig. 3-1. Percentage of total cardiovascular deaths attributable to specific cardio-vascular diseases. (Based on data from Cardiovascular diseases in the United States.[5])

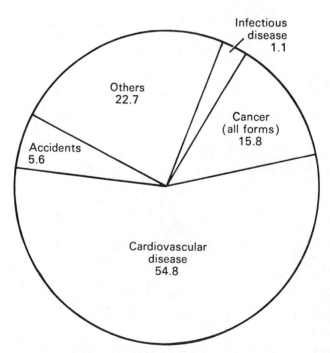

Fig. 3-2. Major causes of death in United States together with percentage of deaths attributable to each of these causes. (Drawing by Eugene Sinervo; based on data from President's Commission on Heart Disease, Cancer and Stroke.[31])

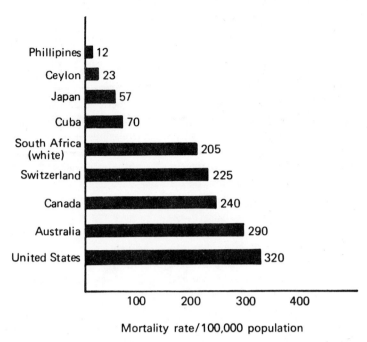

Mortality rate/100,000 population

Fig. 3-3. Mortality rates from atherosclerosis and degenerative heart disease from certain selected countries. (Based on data from Demographic Yearbook, 1967, New York, 1968, Statistical Office of the United Nations.)

The leading causes of death in the United States in 1900 and also in 1965 are listed in Table 3-1.

Reduction of communicable diseases is partly responsible for several changes in the relative importance of these diseases during the last sixty-five years. However, not to be overlooked is the sharp increase in the death rate associated with diseases of the heart, with cancer, and with stroke.

Also of concern is the fact that there has been an increase in the mortality rate from cardiovascular disease among relatively young men. White,[41] for example, indicates that coronary heart disease accounts for 16% of all deaths in the 25- to 35-year age group, 33% in the 35- to 45-year age group, 45% in the 45- to 55-year age group, 53% in the 55- to 65-year age group, and 70% for those 65 years of age or older.

Probably the most alarming factor, however, is that the incidence of death from cardiovascular disease in the United States is higher than in any other country in the world. The annual mortality rates for deaths due to athero-sclerotic heart disease for certain selected countries are presented in Fig. 3-3. These figures are based on the annual mortality rate per 100,000 of the total population, both male and female.

COMMON CARDIOVASCULAR DISEASES
Atherosclerosis

Atherosclerosis is the underlying cause of more than 95% of all cardio-vascular disease. It is the more important form of arteriosclerosis, or hardening of the arteries. With atherosclerosis there is a thickening as well as a hardening of the walls of the arteries. Several lipids are present in the bloodstream, including cholesterol, triglyceride, phospholipids, and fatty acids. It is believed that atherosclerosis usually begins with a deposit of some form of fatty material on the inner layer of the arterial wall. Such a deposit is known as a plaque. After a time these deposits may become embedded within the inner layer of the artery—the intima. The lumen, or opening, through which the blood must pass gradually narrows with each deposit, and the blood flow may be seriously impaired.[10]

Atherosclerosis may begin at an early age, and yet the symptoms may not appear until middle age or later. Sanders[35] indicates that "a fact often over-looked by the public is that almost everyone in the United States over the age of twelve has atherosclerosis to some degree." This appears to be supported in a study by Enos, Holmes, and Beyer,[10] who examined 300 United States soldiers killed in action during the Korean War. The average age of these soldiers was only 22.1 years. Despite this fact it was discovered by means of autopsy that some form of coronary atherosclerosis was present in over 77% of the hearts of these soldiers. The extent of this varied from slight "fibrous" thickening to large plaques causing complete occlusion of one or more of the major vessels of the heart.

A person can have atherosclerosis for 50 or 60 years or more and die from some other cause. However, over 1 million persons in the United States each year are not so fortunate.

Coronary thrombosis

Coronary thrombosis is the medical name for what is commonly referred to by most people as a "heart attack." This occurs when a section of the heart muscle is deprived of its blood supply. The stage is set for the heart attack by the gradual narrowing of the coronary arteries. Most heart attacks are caused when a blood clot, or thrombus, lodges in one of the narrowed coronary arteries—thus limiting the blood supply to a certain area of the heart. Although such an attack may be sudden, it usually is the result of the slowly developing process of atherosclerosis in the coronary arteries. Following is an excellent description of a heart attack given by the American Heart Association:

Mr. B., a business executive in his early fifties, had eaten an unusually hearty dinner after a long hard day at the office, and had retired early. He felt weary but otherwise well. Shortly after midnight he was awakened by a sense of heavy pressure under the sternum. It persisted and grew steadily more severe, although he took soda in hot water. He felt faint and perspired profusely. As the pain became more and more severe he agreed to let his wife call the doctor, who arrived soon after one o'clock. He immediately gave Mr. B. an injection of morphine to ease the pain, but had to repeat this in twenty minutes because the first dose gave no relief.

The patient dozed at intervals for the next five or six hours. Whenever he awoke he was conscious of dull pain in the center of his chest. At about noon he was moved very carefully by ambulance to the hospital, where he was placed in an oxygen tent. This was done partly for his comfort and partly in the hope that the use of oxygen at this early stage of the illness would reduce the size of any scar that might form later in the heart.

Mr. B. was quite tired upon arrival at the hospital, and the discomfort in the chest was troublesome enough to require morphine or similar drugs several times during the next twenty-four hours. On his second day in the hospital he had a slight fever, and this persisted for four days. The pain in the chest was only slight on the second day, and ceased by the evening of that day.

Within a week he felt perfectly well, but his doctor wisely insisted that he remain at almost complete rest for another two or three weeks in order to ensure more complete healing of the injury that had occurred in his heart. Not having been confined to bed for many years, Mr. B. was inclined to rebel at first. But he agreed to follow instructions when the reasons were explained more fully a few days later.

For almost three weeks after his attack, Mr. B. remained in bed. However, he was permitted to use a commode at the bedside for bowel movements. He was encouraged to do gentle leg and foot exercises in his legs. A few days after entering the hospital he was allowed to feed himself. About a week later he was permitted to have a few visitors, and several days after this he began to have occasional conferences with his secretary and business associates.

Mr. B. was given small portions of food during his stay in the hospital, to lessen the demands made upon the heart by digesting heavy meals. The number of calories was also limited, to help bring his weight down.

Toward the end of the third week he was allowed to sit on the edge of his bed for a few minutes several times a day. When he was able to do this without fatigue he was helped into a comfortable chair and permitted to sit up for longer periods each day. As his strength increased, he was encouraged to walk about his room and in the hospital corridor.

Mr. B. was discharged from the hospital a little more than one month after his admission, feeling perfectly well except for slight physical weakness. His doctor encouraged him to increase his stair-climbing and walking, slowly but steadily. Within several weeks he was able to go for rides in his car.

Two months after his attack Mr. B. felt as well as ever, and was eager to resume his regular business life. His physician persuaded him to postpone his return to work for another two weeks, when he was allowed to go to his office for half of each day. By the end of two weeks he was working on his regular schedule again, but was careful to avoid unnecessary physical fatigue as well as those business matters which caused emotional stress. He lost twelve pounds of excess weight and had not smoked cigarettes since the day of his attack. He declared that he felt better than he had in many years.[23]

When part of the heart is deprived of sufficient oxygen, certain damage may occur. This damage is referred to as *myocardial infarction. Myocardium* is the Latin name of the heart muscle. The word *infarction* simply means death of tissue by loss of its normal supply of oxygenated blood. Thus the term *myocardial infarction* indicates that a small portion of the heart muscle has died because an artery or branch of an artery that formerly supplied it with oxygenated blood has been closed.[23]

Symptoms of a heart attack vary from person to person, but the usual symptoms are (1) severe painful sensation in the front of the chest, (2) sweating, (3) shortness of breath, and (4) loss of consciousness.[22]

Stroke

A stroke occurs when a part of the brain is deprived of its blood supply and as a result the nerve cells in that part of the brain cannot function properly. When this happens, the part of the body controlled by these nerve cells cannot function either.[12]

The importance of a regular supply of oxygen to the brain is clearly demonstrated during prolonged vigorous exercise, when the body demands additional oxygen for use by the working muscles. Blood is diverted from various parts of the body to the working musculature. The brain is the only area to which the blood supply does not change, which demonstrates the importance of a steady supply of blood to the brain. The blood supply to the brain may be impaired by clotting, compression, or hemorrhage.[37]

The most common cause of a stroke is a thrombus becoming lodged in one of the arteries leading to the brain. If this occurs, the blood supply to part of the brain is impaired, and the subject has suffered from what is known as cerebral thrombosis. Again, in the case of a stroke, atherosclerosis is an important underlying cause. A stroke also can be caused by a brain tumor or from excess pressure's being placed on the brain or on an artery supplying blood to the brain. A third cause of stroke is bleeding or hemorrhage in an artery supplying blood to the brain. This reduces the supply of blood available to the brain.

Angina pectoris

Angina pectoris is the name given to a chest pain that usually is caused by insufficient blood reaching the heart muscle at times when it is needed. Usually when the demands of the heart cannot be met, it is because of coronary atherosclerosis—the small coronary arteries have become narrowed. Angina pectoris attacks may follow periods of physical exertion or emotional stress. They usually are felt below the sternum, and relief may be obtained by immediate rest.

Hypertension

Hypertension is defined as a condition occurring when blood pressure remains consistently above the normal range. It can result in serious damage to the heart and arteries because the heart is forced to work harder and becomes grossly inefficient. It is a common disorder in this country. Statistics from the most recent National Health Survey indicate that at least 17 million American adults suffer from hypertension.[24] Despite the fact that it occurs so frequently,

medical research still has not determined its exact cause or causes. However, almost all cases of hypertension can be controlled by any of a variety of drugs effective for reducing elevated blood pressure. The death rate from hypertension has decreased by nearly 50% during the last decade as a result of improved diagnosis and treatment.[39]

IDENTIFICATION OF RISK FACTORS

A number of risk factors have been identified through careful study of the living habits and medical records of various segments of the population in this country and through similar studies in other countries. As a result of these studies the following seven factors have been identified as cardiovascular disease risk factors:

1. Increased cholesterol
2. Obesity or excess weight
3. High blood pressure
4. Heavy smoking
5. High level of stress
6. Positive heredity
7. Lack of activity

Any one of these so-called risk factors can increase the likelihood of cardiovascular disease, and a combination of two or more factors multiplies the risk (Fig. 3-4).[31] The following summary, presented by Berg, is based on a long-term study carried out over a period of twenty years in Framingham, Massachusetts.

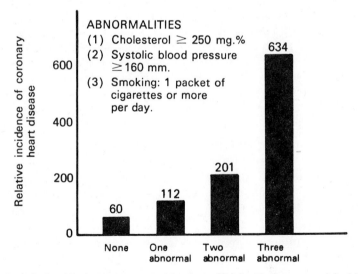

Fig. 3-4. Relationship between a combination of high-risk factors and incidence of coronary heart disease. Note that, if a person has all three abnormalities, his chances are greater than ten times that for someone who has none of the abnormalities. (Based on data from Kannel.[26])

If you have ever wondered what your chances of having a heart attack are, scientists now have the answer. If you are a male, thirty to sixty years old, the odds are one in ten you'll be hit by one before you age another ten years—with one chance in three you will die as a result of it. If you are overweight with high blood pressure and too much cholesterol in your blood, your chances of having a heart attack leap to one in two. And when you add heavy smoking you've blown your chances—you're it. Women rate the same odds as men, but for the ladies the risk begins twenty years later in life. That's the overall message a know-it-all computer is printing out after being fed over a million pieces of data gathered by scientists who have closely watched 5,127 men and women for almost twenty years.[1]

The results from this first long-term project undertaken in this county are alarming, and yet it is not uncommon for a person to disregard them completely and show no concern. It is easier for most people to believe that the disasters of life happen only to others and not to them, and so they take no precautionary measures to avoid these disorders. The director of this study has presented an excellent, up-to-date summary of the situation as it exists in this country today:

> Heart attacks are not natural, they are man-created, and if the knowledge we have now were properly applied we could halve the number of deaths from coronary attacks; in short, we could probably save over 200,000 lives a year.[25]

An excellent summary of the situation as it exists today also is presented by the American Heart Association:

> There is enough evidence to suggest that the living habits of millions of Americans are endangering their hearts at a comparatively early age. These habits usually begin in childhood, with living patterns learned from parents. . . . By the time they reach their thirties and forties, too many Americans are overweight, lead physically inactive lives and smoke heavily. Many have high levels of cholesterol and other fatty substances in their blood. The detection of major risks is one of the most encouraging advances of medical knowledge for it points to precautions we can all take to increase our chances of living longer and enjoying good health.[32]

Thus it appears to be important to examine carefully the available information that relates to each of the risk factors that have been identified. By examining this information, the relative importance of each risk factor can be determined, and this information may aid the individual in understanding future scientific developments in this area. The ultimate aim, of course, is to have people understand exactly what they must do to reduce their chances of suffering from cardiovascular diseases and to have them take these precautionary measures.

FACTORS ASSOCIATED WITH CARDIOVASCULAR DISEASE
Increased cholesterol level in the bloodstream

Cholesterol is a fatlike substance, a certain amount of which must always be present in the body to maintain life and good health. However, excess amounts of cholesterol are detrimental to one's health, since high cholesterol levels have been shown to be associated with the development of certain heart and blood vessel diseases. A certain amount of cholesterol is manufactured by the body itself, but there also are large quantities contained in certain foods. Foods that are rich in natural cholesterol are the dangerous ones. These usually are referred to as saturated fats. Fats are made up of carbon and hydrogen molecules. If each carbon molecule is combined with two hydrogen molecules, the combination is referred to as a saturated fat. When there are fewer than two hydrogen molecules for each carbon molecule, they are referred to as either monounsaturated or polyunsaturated, depending on the number of carbon molecules that are not combined with two hydrogen molecules.[4] A listing of the cholesterol content of some common foods is included in Table 3-2.

In the average American diet approximately 40% of the total calories consumed are derived from fat. This is a much higher percentage than in other countries. In Japan, for example, fat comprises less than 10% of the total diet. When the average, or normal, cholesterol levels of these two countries are compared, it can be seen that these values reflect the type of food that is eaten. In the United States, where the amount of fat consumed is much higher than in Japan, the cholesterol level that is considered normal also is much higher. The range of cholesterol that is considered normal in the United States is 220 to 240 mg/100 ml. In the Framingham study, for example, the average serum cholesterol level in adult males tested was 220 mg/100 ml with less than 5%

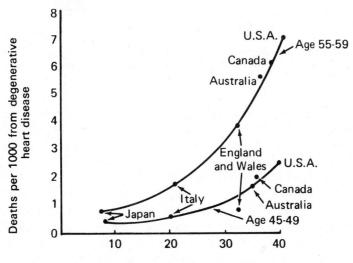

Fig. 3-5. Relationship between intake of calories from fat and death from degenerative heart disease in six selected countries. Note that in those countries where there was a high level of fat intake, there was also a high incidence of degenerative heart disease. (Adapted from Keys.[27])

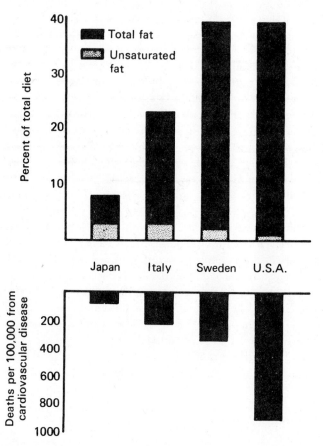

Fig. 3-6. Comparison between the amount and type of fat in the diet of four countries and the death rates due to cardiovascular heart disease. (Adapted from Cant.[4])

of the population having values of less than 160 mg/100 ml.[7] In Japan, however, the average cholesterol level has been found to be only 150 mg/100 ml.[1]

Several studies have attempted to examine the relationship between the amount of fat in the diet and the incidence of death from cardiovascular disease. Results of two of these studies are presented in Figs. 3-5 and 3-6. This can be considered only as indirect evidence, and one must be careful in interpreting these results. They merely suggest a relationship between the two variables; and certainly, no matter how plausible such an association may appear, it is not in itself proof of a cause-effect relationship. One must study all the available information and then draw a conclusion based on the information.

Various studies show that when the population is divided into groups according to levels of cholesterol, the higher the level of cholesterol, the higher the incidence of cardiovascular disease. The data obtained from the Framing-

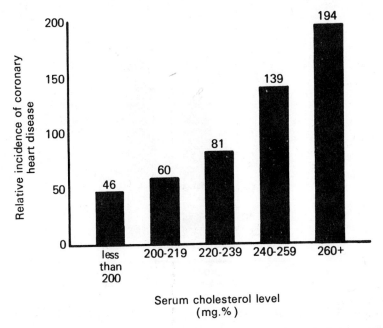

Fig. 3-7. Risk of developing coronary heart disease according to cholesterol levels. (Adapted from Dawber and Kannel.[7])

ham study* clearly show this relationship. These data are presented in Fig. 3-7. It can be seen that when the cholesterol level was less than 200 mg/100 ml the incidence of cardiovascular disease was less than half that of the total population. In this group in which the cholesterol level was 260 mg/100 ml or more, the rate was almost twice that of the entire group examined. It was therefore over four times as great in the latter group as in the group that had a cholesterol level of less than 200 mg/100 ml.[5]

Results similar to these have been found by Gertler and White.[17] They compared subjects who had experienced some type of cardiovascular disease with similar subjects who had no history of cardiovascular disease. Their results are summarized in Fig. 3-8. Again it can clearly be seen that the group with the history of cardiovascular disease had a much higher mean cholesterol level (286 mg/100 ml) than the group with no history of cardiovascular disease (224 mg/100 ml).

---

*The Framingham study was the first organized long-term study undertaken in this county to examine certain cardiovascular risk factors. It involved over 5000 men and women from the city of Framingham, Massachusetts, and was conducted over a twenty-year period by medical personnel. The results of this study will be referred to throughout this chapter, since up-to-date information has been obtained relative to cardiovascular disease.

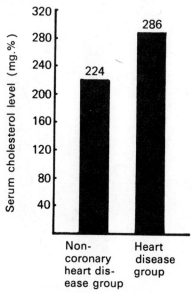

Fig. 3-8. Serum cholesterol levels in coronary and noncoronary heart disease subjects. (Based on data from Gertler and White.[18])

Table 3-2. Cholesterol content of certain foods high in cholesterol content

Food	Approximate weight of serving (ounces)	Milligrams cholesterol per serving	Food	Approximate weight of serving (ounces)	Milligrams cholesterol per serving
Beef	3	63	Shrimp	2	76
Pork	3	63	Lobster	2	120
Lamb	3	63	Oysters	2	120
Veal	3	81	Liver	2	180
Fish	3	63	Egg (whole)	1½	275
Chicken	3	54	Tuna	3½	60
Cottage cheese	2	10	Turkey	3	60
Crab	2	76	Margarine	3	65

It should be emphasized that there is actually no cholesterol level at which the incidence of cardiovascular disease takes a sudden rise, but there is general agreement that the lower the cholesterol level, the lower the risk of suffering some form of cardiovascular disease.

The American Heart Association presents three dietary recommendations for those who wish to reduce their chances of cardiovascular disease:

1. A caloric intake adjusted to achieve and maintain the proper weight

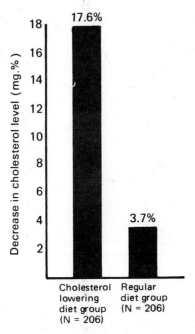

Fig. 3-9. Effect of a special low-cholesterol diet on the serum cholesterol level. Note that the decrease in the cholesterol level of the special diet group is approximately five times that of the regular diet group. (Based on data from Leren.[28])

2. A total intake of less than 40% of the total calories from fat, with the ratio of polyunsaturated fat to saturated fat approximately 2:1
3. A substantial reduction of cholesterol in the diet to less than 300 mg daily[8]

Present studies have shown that the level of cholesterol in the blood is reduced considerably when these recommendations are followed. For example, Page and Brown,[30] using fifty-five volunteer subjects over a 10-month period, were able to reduce the cholesterol level 14% by reducing the amount of saturated fat in the diet. Not only was there a drop in the cholesterol level, but there also was a corresponding fall in the diastolic blood pressure and in body weight. Leren[28] was able to show that not only is there a reduction in the cholesterol level with a controlled cholesterol-lowering diet, but that this also is associated with a lower incidence of cardiovascular disease. This study conducted in Oslo, Norway, involved 412 males ranging from 30 to 64 years of age. Each subject involved had survived a previous experience of myocardial infarction. These 412 subjects were randomly assigned to one of two groups. One group was placed on a cholesterol-lowering diet while the other group continued on its regular diet. The reduction of cholesterol in the diet group was 17.6% as compared to 3.7% in the control group. These results are graphically represented in Fig. 3-9.

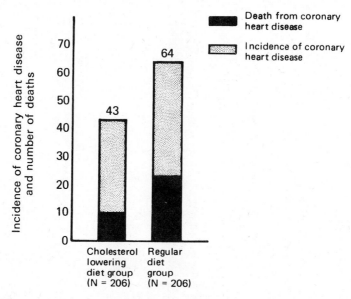

Fig. 3-10. Relationship between cholesterol intake and the incidence of coronary heart disease and death from coronary heart disease. (Based on data from Leren.[28])

Table 3-3. Summary of serum cholesterol changes and associated incidence of coronary heart disease

	Experimental group	Control group
Number of subjects	94	61
Mean serum cholesterol level	236 mg/100 ml	252 mg/100 ml
Mean cholesterol level after 6 weeks	214 mg/100 ml	259 mg/100 ml
Mean cholesterol change	–22 mg/100 ml	+7 mg/100 ml
Total cases of new coronary heart disease	17	30

Of the 206 subjects in the diet-controlled group, only 43 suffered a subsequent myocardial infarction, and of these 43 attacks, only 10 were fatal in the five years that these subjects were observed. Sixty-four subjects in the control group suffered a subsequent myocardial infarction, and of these 64, 23 were fatal. These results are presented in Fig. 3-10.

Findings consistent with these were obtained by Turpeinen et al.[38] in a similar study. The results of this study are summarized in Table 3-3.

These studies indicate that when the amount of cholesterol in the diet is lowered, the serum cholesterol level is reduced, and that there is a corresponding reduction in the incidence of coronary heart disease associated with such a change.

In summary, it should be emphasized that coronary heart disease is a result of many factors. A diet that is rich in saturated fat and cholesterol is one important risk factor. Such a diet can safely be modified, and such a modification has been shown to be associated with a corresponding reduction in the incidence of coronary heart disease.

Obesity or excess weight

Obesity may be defined as an excessive accumulation of body fat. According to Kannel,[25] it has been shown to have a definite relationship to certain cardiovascular diseases, possibly due to the following:

1. Extra stress is placed on the heart because of the added work load.
2. Obesity is closely associated with increased blood pressure.
3. With obesity there is usually an increased level of cholesterol and other lipids.

Thus it would appear advantageous to reduce the amount of body fat or excess body weight in view of the favorable effect this would have on the other related factors. In the Framingham study, subjects who were 20 pounds or more overweight suffered three times as many fatal heart attacks as those who could be considered of normal weight.

High blood pressure

Another risk factor that has clearly been identified with cardiovascular disease is high blood pressure. It has been demonstrated that with an elevated blood pressure level the process of atherosclerosis is accelerated, and there is a corresponding increase in cardiovascular disease. The results of the Framingham study clearly demonstrate this relationship (Fig. 3-11). It can be seen from this information that the higher the systolic blood pressure level, the greater the risk of developing coronary heart disease. This incidence of heart disease in those subjects who experienced a systolic blood pressure of 180 mm or more was almost eight times as great as the group having a systolic blood pressure of less than 120 mm.[7]

Heavy smoking

In a recent article the American Heart Association reviewed the relationship between heavy smoking and the incidence of cardiovascular disease. The following summary was presented:

A number of medical studies have been made, nearly all demonstrating a statistical association between heavy cigarette smoking and death or illness from coronary heart disease. In these studies, death rates from coronary heart disease in middle-aged men were found to be from fifty to one hundred and fifty percent higher among heavy cigarette smokers than among those who do not smoke. This statistical association does not prove that heavy cigarette smoking causes coronary heart disease, but the data strongly suggest that heavy cigarette smoking may contribute to or accelerate the development of coronary heart disease or its complications.[6]

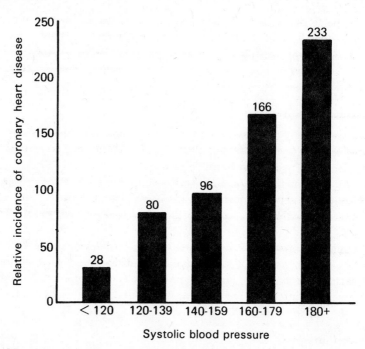

Fig. 3-11. Risk of developing coronary heart disease according to systolic blood pressure levels. (Adapted from Dawber and Kannel.[7])

Table 3-4. Comparison of smokers and nonsmokers with regard to the incidence of death from all causes and death from coronary heart disease

Group	Number	Deaths from coronary heart disease	Ratio	Deaths from all causes	Ratio
Nonsmokers	812	17	2.6	13	2.0
Cigarette smokers	1,272	92	9.0	64	6.3

After examination of some of the evidence available, each person should draw his own conclusions concerning this important matter.

In a report in *The Journal of the American Medical Association*, Doyle et al.[9] compared the results of two long-term research studies designed to examine the relationship between cardiovascular disease and cigarette smoking. One of these studies was conducted in Albany, New York, and involved 2,084 male subjects ranging from 39 to 55 years of age. These men were studied over an eight-year period, and the incidence of heart disease was related to their smoking habits. The findings of this study indicated that those men who reported smoking twenty or more cigarettes a day experienced a much higher rate of heart disease. The risk was slightly more than three times as great in

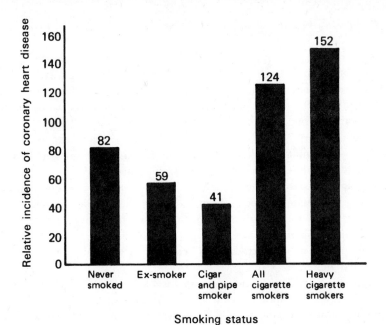

Fig. 3-12. Relationship between smoking and incidence of coronary heart disease. (Adapted from Kannel.[26])

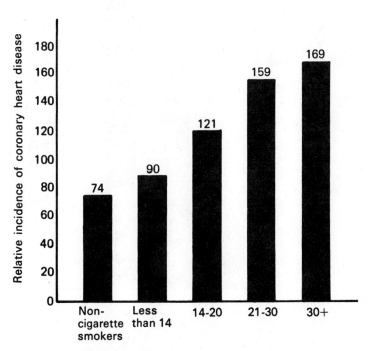

Fig. 3-13. Relationship between number of cigarettes smoked and incidence of coronary heart disease. Note that the incidence of coronary heart disease increased as the number of cigarettes smoked increased. (Adapted from Kannel.[26])

this group as in the nonsmoking group. These results are presented in Table 3-4. This study also indicates that the ratio of deaths from all causes among the cigarette smokers was slightly more than three times that of the nonsmokers.

The results of the study conducted in Albany, New York, were compared to those obtained from the Framingham study of 2,282 men. These men ranged from 30 to 62 years of age and were observed over a ten-year period. The results of the Framingham study relating to smoking are presented in Figs. 3-12 and 3-13. These results can be summarized as follows:

1. The incidence of coronary heart disease among heavy smokers (152) was approximately twice as great as among the nonsmokers (82).
2. There was a surprisingly small incidence of heart disease among cigar and pipe smokers (41).
3. The incidence of heart disease increased as the numbers of cigarettes smoked increased.
4. After an individual stops smoking, his risk quickly reverts to the low-risk level of those individuals who never have smoked.

Another finding relating to this study was that the incidence of smoking

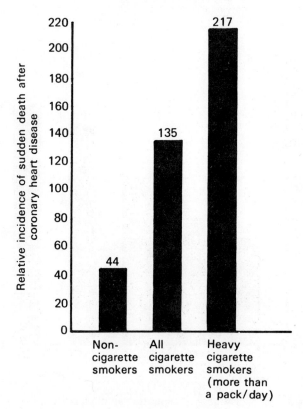

Fig. 3-14. Relationship of cigarette smoking to sudden death, immediately following coronary heart disease. (Adapted from Kannel.[26])

appeared to be related to the prevalence of sudden death (Fig. 3-14). It can clearly be seen that the risk of sudden death was approximately five times as great in the heavy smokers (217) as in the nonsmokers (44).[26]

The comparison of these two long-term studies revealed similar findings in each case despite the fact that the studies were conducted in two different states.

A larger project, involving 187,766 men from ten different states, was organized by Hammond and Horn.[19-21] These men were studied for 44 months in an attempt to determine whether smoking influenced the overall death rate and, if so, which diseases were involved.

They found that a total of 4,406 deaths occurred among those with a history of regular cigarette smoking. This was 1,783 more than would have occurred had the rate been the same as it was in the nonsmoking group (Fig. 3-15). The study also revealed that of these excess deaths among cigarette smokers approximately 25% could be attributed to excess deaths from cancer and approximately 50% to excess deaths from coronary heart disease.

The relationship between the incidence of death from coronary heart dis-

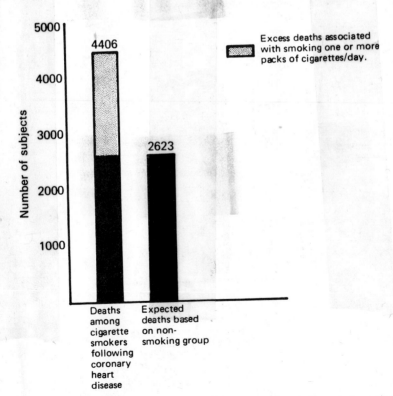

Fig. 3-15. Number of deaths associated with coronary heart disease among smokers and nonsmokers. (Based on data from Hammond and Horn.[19])

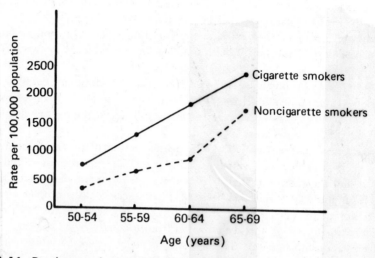

Fig. 3-16. Death rates from coronary heart disease according to smoking history and by age. (Adapted from Hammond and Horn.[19])

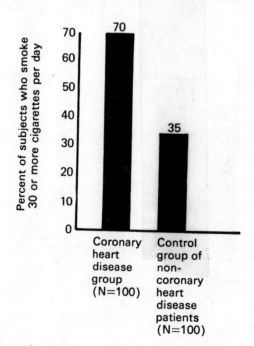

Fig. 3-17. Incidence of heavy cigarette smoking in a coronary heart disease group and a noncoronary heart disease group. (Based on data from Russek.[33])

ease and the status of cigarette smoking is presented in Fig. 3-16. Again it can clearly be seen that there are approximately twice as many deaths among those who smoke at least a pack of cigarettes or more a day than among those who do not smoke.

Russek[33] presents information of a slightly different nature relating to smoking and heart disease. In his study a group of subjects who had experienced some form of heart disease was compared with a control group of subjects who had no previous heart disease history. It was found that 70% of the heart disease group smoked thirty or more cigarettes a day, whereas only 35% of the control group were classified as smokers, using the same criteria (Fig. 3-17).

In summary, with regard to smoking there appears to be the following agreement:

1. Men with a history of regular cigarette smoking have a considerably higher death rate than men who do not smoke or men who smoke cigars or pipes.
2. Men who stop smoking quickly reduce their risk factor to the level of those who do not smoke.
3. Men who smoke regularly have a much higher incidence of coronary disease than men who do not smoke.
4. The higher the number of cigarettes smoked daily, the higher the incidence of heart disease and the higher the incidence of sudden death.

These statistical studies almost unanimously indicate that smoking is a very important factor as far as coronary heart disease is concerned and that significantly less risk is encountered by nonsmokers and by those who stop smoking.

High level of stress

Stress is defined as "the physical or emotional factor that causes bodily or mental tension."[40] There are many causal factors determining the level of stress. When these occur, the body is able to overcome the stressor or else there is an increased level of anxiety or tension created within the body. Selye[36] indicates that when an organism is exposed to a stressor, the response is in the form of a general reaction that includes three phases: (1) an alarm reaction, (2) a stage of resistance, and (3) a stage of exhaustion. He further indicates that in some instances the body can prepare for future stress by gradual adaptation to a stressor in small doses.

Much stress may be caused by an individual's occupation. This is referred to as occupationally related stress and is probably the most significant type. Friedman and Rosenman[15] have developed a set of criteria for evaluating a person's stress level. They indicate that a person can be classified into one of two groups. The first of these groups is referred to as type A, which consists of individuals exhibiting a high stress level and rating high on the following criteria:

1. *Ambition*—an intense, sustained drive to achieve self-selected but usually poorly defined goals.

2. *Competitiveness*—profound inclination and eagerness to compete.
3. *Aggressiveness*—persistent desire for recognition and advancement.
4. *Profound sense of time urgency*—continuous involvement in multiple functions while constantly subject to restrictions.
5. *Drive*—persistent efforts to accelerate the rate of execution of many physical and mental functions.

These traits are normally present in most individuals, but in the type A person they are present to an excessive degree. Individuals who fall in this group include those who cannot stand to have unscheduled time on their hands and who become very upset when they are kept waiting.

Those who rate low in these traits were classified as type B. This is the type of person who usually is able to relax easily. Very seldom does he let outside factors adversely influence his emotional state. The level of anxiety and tension of a type B person is therefore very low.

In an attempt to determine the relationship between stress level and cardiovascular disease Friedman and Rosenman[15] compared a group of type A subjects with a group of type B subjects with regard to certain factors relating to heart disease. Each group contained eighty-three subjects selected so that they did not differ with regard to age, height, weight, total caloric intake, total fat intake, and amount of physical activity. There was a large difference between the two groups with regard to the incidence of coronary heart disease (Fig. 3-18). This was seven times more prevalent in the high stress group than in the low stress group.

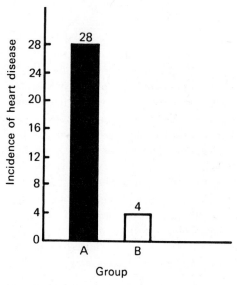

Fig. 3-18. Comparison of Group A (high stress) and Group D (low stress) with regard to incidence of coronary heart disease (age range 30 to 59 years). (Based on data from Friedman and Rosenman.[15])

The two groups also differed significantly in the amount of cholesterol in the bloodstream (Fig. 3-19). The mean cholesterol level in the high stress group was 253 mg/100 ml compared to 215 mg/100 ml in the low stress group.

A later study indicated that subjects who were classified as type A experienced difficulty in clearing fat from the bloodstream after ingestion of a high-fat meal.[16] This explains the high cholesterol level found in the subjects.

Additional studies that relate the amount of stress to the incidence of heart disease are available. Russek and Zohman[34] compared a group of coronary heart disease patients with a control group that had not experienced any form of cardiovascular disease. Each group consisted of 100 subjects ranging from 25 to 40 years of age. The results pertaining to occupational stress (Fig. 3-20) clearly show that the amount of stress experienced by the coronary group was much higher than that of the noncoronary group. They also found that in the coronary group 25% held more than one job, 60% put in more than 60 hours of work per week, and 20% experienced unusual fear and discomfort associated with their work.

Russek[33] collected data from 4,981 male subjects ranging from 40 to 69 years of age. He grouped these subjects into three categories relating to stress —low, medium, and high—and examined the incidence of heart disease as it related to the stress level. His findings (Fig. 3-21) clearly indicate that the higher the level of stress, the greater the incidence of coronary heart disease.

He also examined the relationship between stress level and incidence of cigarette smoking. These results are presented in Fig. 3-22. This study indicates

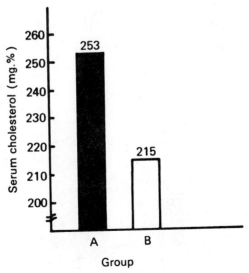

Fig. 3-19. Comparison of Group A (high stress) and Group B (low stress) with regard to level of serum cholesterol (age range 30 to 59 years). (Based on data from Friedman and Rosenman.[15])

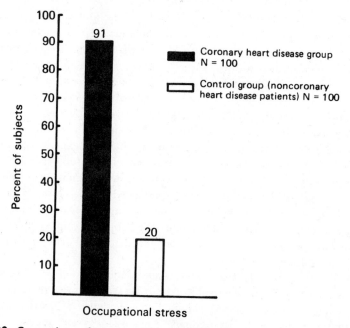

Fig. 3-20. Comparison of a coronary heart disease group and a noncoronary heart disease control group with regard to the incidence of occupational stress (age range 25 to 40 years). (Based on data from Russek and Zohman.[34])

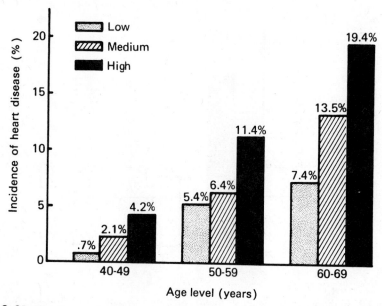

Fig. 3-21. Incidence of coronary heart disease according to stress level (low, medium, and high) and age. (Adapted from Russek.[33])

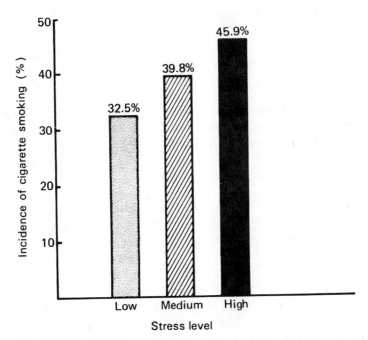

Fig. 3-22. Incidence of cigarette smoking as related to level of stress. (Adapted from Russek.[33])

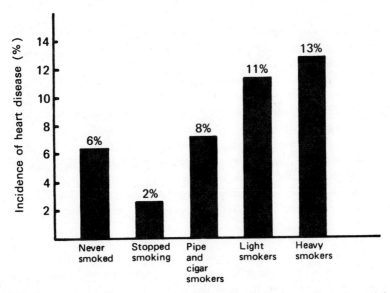

Fig. 3-23. Incidence of coronary heart disease according to smoking habits. (Adapted from Russek.[33])

that smoking patterns in the individual or group may provide an index by which emotional tensions may be relatively assessed.

His findings relative to coronary heart disease and the incidence of smoking (Fig. 3-23) are in agreement with the findings previously discussed.

Positive heredity

The incidence of coronary heart disease appears to be greater among those who have a history of heart disease in the immediate family than among those who have no history of heart disease. The results of a study by Gertler et al.[17] are presented in Fig. 3-24, *A*, and those obtained by Russek and Zohman,[34] in Fig. 3-24, *B*. Both studies indicate that a subject is more likely to suffer some form of cardiovascular disease if he comes from a family with a history of heart disease. Persons who fit into this category certainly cannot do anything about choosing their parents, but they should show much more concern about reducing the other risk factors about which they can do something.

Lack of physical activity

In the previous discussion on physical fitness, the sedentary life pattern that exists in this country was emphasized. It was shown that automation, elevators, television sets, and many other mechanical devices have reduced the expenditure of physical effort. With this reduction of physical activity in modern living there has been a concurrent increase not only in the incidence of cardiovascular disease but also in the associated mortality rate.

One cannot prove a causal relationship between the decrease in activity and the increase in cardiovascular disease. There is, however, a growing body of knowledge suggesting that physical inactivity may be one of many possible factors involved in the increasing incidence of coronary heart disease.[13]

Many studies indicate that a sedentary life increases the chances of suffering a heart attack. Most of these studies compare the incidence of heart disease associated with an active occupation with that associated with a relatively inactive type of occupation. One of the earliest studies was conducted by Morris.[29] His findings showed that the incidence of heart disease was twice as great among English bus drivers (least active) as among the bus conductors (most active). He showed that bus drivers and conductors had the same social background and that their living conditions were highly similar. The bus conductor working on double-deck buses walks up and down the stairs a great deal and is on his feet practically all the time during the working day. The driver during the same period remains seated and has limited opportunity to move around.

Because of certain uncontrolled factors in this study, Morris and his co-workers extended it to include subjects from many walks of life. In all, some 31,000 subjects were examined, including post office employees, farmers, laborers, and a number of professional groups. Similar results were obtained in these studies. Heart disease occurred almost twice as frequently among telephone operators as among postmen. The telephone operator sits at his

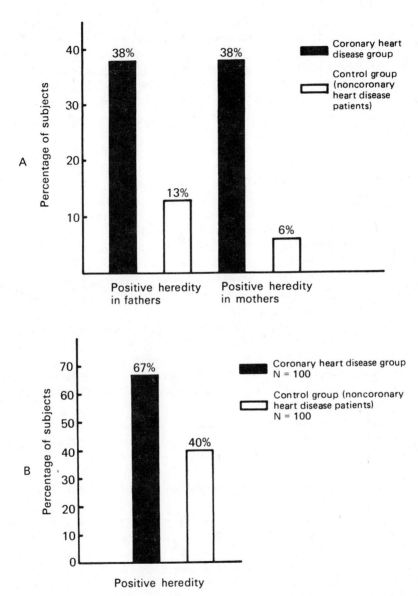

Fig. 3-24. A, Comparison of percentage of subjects with a family history of cardio-vascular disease in a coronary and a noncoronary control group. **B,** Comparison of percentage of subjects with a family history of cardiovascular disease in a coronary and a noncoronary control group. Note that in the group suffering from some form of coronary heart disease is a much higher history of heart disease (67%) compared to the noncoronary group (40%). (**A** based on data from Gertler et al.[12]; **B** based on data from Russek and Zohman.[34])

desk during the entire work day, whereas the postman is very active as he carries mail and delivers it.[29]

In other kinds of occupations similar differences were shown to exist. In each case, the incidence of heart disease was lower in those whose occupation involved a high level of physical work. The incidence of heart diesase was highest in each case in the least active occupations. Morris concluded that lack of exercise and a sedentary way of life predispose a person to heart disease. His advice to the middle-aged person was not to give up physical activity and adopt a wholly sedentary way of life, since this would increase his chance of being a victim of heart attack.

Brunner and Manelis[3] studied the relationship between the incidence of heart disease and the physical activity level. They used almost 9,000 men and women ranging from 30 to 55 years of age. This study was undertaken in Israel, where all the subjects lived in communal settlements. These subjects were therefore ethnically homogeneous and the environmental conditions— such as standard of living, diet, housing, cultural activity, and recreation— were virtually uniform. It was thus possible to control many factors that other investigators were unable to take into consideration. Results showed that the incidence of heart disease was more than three times greater among the in- active subjects than among the active group. The mortality rate also was three times greater in the sedentary group.

In a more recent study, Brunner[2] obtained almost identical results. He used over 10,000 men and women ranging in age from 40 to 64 years. All these subjects, again, lived in collective settlements in Israel under uniform environmental conditions. The incidence of some form of cardiovascular dis- ease was from two and one-half to four times higher in sedentary workers than in nonsedentary workers.

These and many other studies indicate that persons in physically active jobs have a much lower incidence of coronary heart disease than persons in phys- ically inactive jobs.

It also has been shown in several studies that the level of activity is closely associated with the early mortality rate following an initial heart attack. Data obtained by Frank et al.[14] are presented in Fig. 3-25. The mortality rate was found to be almost three times as great in the subjects classified as least active (49%) as that obtained for the most active subjects (17%).

Similar results were obtained by Brunner.[2] He followed carefully for 6 years 282 subjects who experienced an initial heart attack. He found that in the first four weeks after the attack 4.2% of the active workers died, whereas 22.6% of the sedentary workers died. After 6 years 23.1% of the active work- ers had died, whereas 59% of the inactive group had died. (See Fig. 3-26.)

SUMMARY

Seven risk factors associated with a higher incidence of cardiovascular disease have been presented, and evidence from associated research has been discussed. It should be stressed that in no instance can a cause-effect relation-

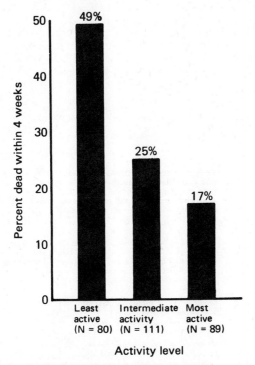

Fig. 3-25. Relationship between death associated with coronary heart disease and level of activity. Note the higher incidence in the death rate among the least active group. (Adapted from Frank et al.[14])

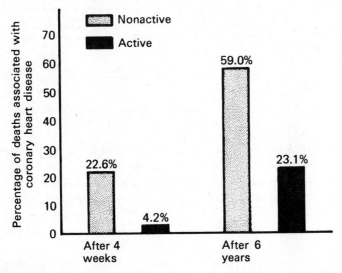

Fig. 3-26. Death rates associated with coronary heart disease, according to activity level. (Adapted from Brunner.[2])

RISKO

The purpose of this game is to give you an estimate of your chances of suffering heart attack.

The game is played by making squares which — from left to right — represent an increase in your RISK FACTORS. These are medical conditions and habits associated with an increased danger of heart attack. Not all risk factors are measurable enough to be included in this game;

RULES:

Study each RISK FACTOR AND its row. Find the box applicable to you and circle the large number in it. For example, if you are 37, circle the number in the box labeled 31-40.
After checking out all the rows, add the circled numbers. This total — your score — is an estimate of your risk.

IF YOU SCORE:

6-11 — Risk well below average
12-17 — Risk below average
18-24 — Risk generally average
25-31 — Risk moderate
32-40 — Risk at a dangerous level
41-62 — Danger urgent. See your doctor now.

HEREDITY:

Count parents, grand-parents, brothers, and sisters who have had heart attack and/or stroke.

TOBACCO SMOKING:

If you inhale deeply and smoke a cigarette way down, add one to your classification. Do NOT subtract because you think you do not inhale or smoke only a half inch on a cigarette.

EXERCISE:

Lower your score one point if you exercise regularly and frequently.

CHOLESTEROL OR SATURATED FAT INTAKE LEVEL:

A cholesterol blood level is best. If you can't get one from your doctor, then estimate honestly the percentage of solid fats you eat. These are usually of animal origin — lard, cream, butter, and beef and lamb fat. If you eat much of this, your cholesterol level probably will be high. The U.S. average, 40%, is too high for good health.

BLOOD PRESSURE:

If you have no recent reading but have passed an insurance or industrial examination chances are you are 140 or less.

SEX:

This line takes into account the fact that men have from 6 to 10 times more heart attacks than women of child bearing age.

ship be established between one or all of these factors and the occurrence of a heart attack; however, the evidence does appear to be conclusive that a person can reduce his chances of suffering a heart attack by taking positive action concerning several of these risk factors. As was quoted previously, "If the knowledge we have now were properly applied we could halve the number of deaths from coronary attacks; in short, we could probably save over 200,000 lives a year."[25]

Students can be made aware of ways in which they can reduce their chances of suffering from some form of cardiovascular disease. In the game called RISKO, developed by the Michigan Heart Association, one

	1	2	3	4	6	8
AGE	10 to 20	21 to 30	31 to 40	41 to 50	51 to 60	61 to 70 and over
HEREDITY	No known history of heart disease	1 relative with cardiovascular disease Over 60	2 relatives with cardiovascular disease Over 60	1 relative with cardiovascular disease Under 60	2 relatives with cardiovascular disease Under 60	3 relatives with cardiovascular disease Under 60
WEIGHT	More than 5 lbs. below standard weight	−5 to +5 lbs. standard weight	6-20 lbs. over weight	21-35 lbs. over weight	36-50 lbs. over weight	51-65 lbs. over weight
TOBACCO SMOKING	Non-user	Cigar and/or pipe	10 cigarettes or less a day	20 cigarettes a day	30 cigarettes a day	40 cigarettes a day or more
EXERCISE	Intensive occupational and recreational exertion	Moderate occupational and recreational exertion	Sedentary work and intense recreational exertion	Sedentary occupational and moderate recreational exertion	Sedentary work and light recreational exertion	Complete lack of all exercise
CHOLES-TEROL OR FAT % IN DIET	Cholesterol below 180 mg.% Diet contains no animal or solid fats	Cholesterol 181-205 mg.% Diet contains 10% animal or solid fats	Cholesterol 206-230 mg.% Diet contains 20% animal or solid fats	Cholesterol 231-255 mg.% Diet contains 30% animal or solid fats	Cholesterol 256-280 mg.% Diet contains 40% animal or solid fats	Cholesterol 281-300 mg.% Diet contains 50% animal or solid fats
BLOOD PRESSURE	100 upper reading	120 upper reading	140 upper reading	160 upper reading	180 upper reading	200 or over upper reading
SEX	Female under 40	Female 40-50	Female over 50	Male	Stocky male	Bald stocky male

can estimate his chances of suffering a heart attack. Read the instructions carefully and determine which category you are classified in.

REFERENCES

1. Berg, R. H.: No more heart attacks, Look, Feb. 2, 1969, p. 32.
2. Brunner, D.: The influence of physical activity on incidence and prognosis of ischemic heart disease. In Raab, W., editor: Prevention of ischemic heart disease, Springfield, Ill., 1966, Charles C Thomas, Publisher, p. 236.
3. Brunner, D., and Manelis, G.: Myocardial infarction among members of communal settlements in Israel, Lancet 2:1049, 1960.

4. Cant, G.: What you must know about diet. In The healthy life, New York, 1966, Time, Inc., pp. 64-71.
5. Cardiovascular diseases in the United States—facts and figures, New York, 1965, American Heart Association, p. 6.
6. Cigarette smoking and cardiovascular disease, New York, 1968, American Heart Association.
7. Dawber, T. R., and Kannel, W. B.: Susceptibility to coronary artery disease, Modern Concepts of Cardiovascular Disease **30**:671-673, July, 1961.
8. Diet and heart disease, New York, 1968, American Heart Association, p. 3.
9. Doyle, J. T., Dawber, T. R., and Kannel, W. B.: The relationship of cigarette smoking to coronary heart disease, The Journal of the American Medical Association **190**:886, Dec., 1964.
10. Enos, W. F., Holmes, R. H., and Beyer, J.: Coronary disease among United States soldiers killed in action in Korea, The Journal of the American Medical Association **152**:1090, 1953.
11. Facts about heart and blood vessel disease, New York, 1966, American Heart Association, p. 3.
12. Facts about strokes, New York, 1964, American Heart Association, p. 2.
13. Fox, S., and Skinner, J.: Physical activity and cardiovascular health, American. Journal of Cardiology **14**:731, Dec., 1964.
14. Frank, C. W., Wainblatt, E., Shapiro, S., et al.: Physical inactivity as a lethal factor in myocardial infarction among men, Circulation **34**:1022, Dec., 1966.
15. Friedman, M., and Rosenman, R. H.: Association of specific overt behaviour with blood and cardiovascular findings, The Journal of the American Medical Association **169**:286, March 21, 1959.
16. Friedman, M., Rosenman, R. H., and Beyers, S. O.: Changes in serum lipids and conjunctional circulation after fat ingestion in men exhibiting a behaviour pattern type A associated with a high incidence of clinical coronary artery disease, Circulation **28**:861, 1963.
17. Gertler, M. M., White, P. D., Cady, L. D., et al.: Coronary heart disease, American Journal of the Medical Sciences **248**:377, 1964.
18. Gertler, M. M., and White, P. D.: Coronary heart disease in young adults, Cambridge, Mass., 1954, Commonwealth Fund.
19. Hammond, E. C., and Horn, D.: The relationship between smoking habits and death rates, The Journal of the American Medical Association **155**:1316, Aug. 7, 1954.
20. Hammond, E. C., and Horn, D.: Smoking and death rates. Report on forty-four months of follow-up of men, The Journal of the American Medical Association **166**:1159, March 8, 1958.
21. Hammond, E. C., and Horn, D.: Death rates by cause, The Journal of the American Medical Association **166**:1294, March 15, 1958.
22. Heart attack, New York, 1956, American Heart Association, p. 3.
23. Heart disease caused by coronary atherosclerosis, New York, 1962, American Heart Association, pp. 3-5.
24. High blood pressure, New York, 1966, American Heart Association, p. 2.
25. Kannel, W. Cited in Berg, R. H.: No more heart attacks, Look, Feb. 2, 1969, p. 30.
26. Kannel, W.: Habits and coronary heart disease. The Framingham heart study, Public Health Service publication no. 1515, Bethesda, Md., 1968, U.S. Department of Health, Education and Welfare, p. 4.

27. Keys, A.: Diet and epidemiology of heart disease, The Journal of the American Medical Association **164:**1912, 1957.
28. Leren, P.: The effect of plasma cholesterol lowering diet in male survivors of myocardial infarction, Acta Medica Scandinavica **466**(supp.):1, 1966.
29. Morris, J. N. et al.: Coronary heart disease and physical activity of work, Lancet **2:**1053, 1953.
30. Page, I. H., and Brown, H. B.: Some observations on the national diet heart study, Circulation **37:**313, March, 1968.
31. President's Commission on Heart Disease, Cancer, and Stroke: A national program to conquer heart disease, cancer, and stroke, Feb. 1965, pp. 26-29.
32. Reduce your risk of heart attack, New York, 1966, American Heart Association, p. 5.
33. Russek, H. I.: Emotional stress, tobacco smoking, and ischemic heart disease. In Raab, W., editor: Prevention of ischemic heart disease, Springfield, Ill., 1966, Charles C Thomas, Publisher, p. 190.
34. Russek, H. I., and Zohman, B. L.: Relative significance of heredity, diet and occupational stress in coronary heart disease in young adults, American Journal of the Medical Sciences **235:**266, 1958.
35. Sanders, H. J.: Heart disease. In Jones, H. L., editor: Science and theory of health, Dubuque, Iowa, 1966, Wm. C. Brown Company, Publishers, p. 235.
36. Selye, H.: The stress of life, New York, 1956, Blakiston Division, McGraw-Hill Book Co., Inc.
37. Strokes—agenda for the family, New York, 1958, American Heart Association, pp. 5-8.
38. Turpeinen, O., Meittinen, M., Karvonen, M. J., et al.: Dietary prevention of coronary heart disease: long term experiment, American Journal of Clinical Nutrition **21:**255, April, 1968.
39. United States Department of Health, Education and Welfare: Hypertension, Washington, D.C., 1969, National Institutes of Health, no. 1714, p. 1.
40. Webster's seventh new collegiate dictionary, Springfield, Mass., 1965, G. & C. Merriam Company, p. 868.
41. White, P. D.: Atherosclerotic heart disease. Paper presented at the annual American Association for Health, Physical Education, and Recreation Convention, Boston, April 11, 1969.

ADDITIONAL READINGS

American Heart Association: Risk factors and coronary disease, New York, Dec., 1968.
Kraus, H., and Raab, W.: Hypokinetic disease, Springfield, Ill., 1961, Charles C Thomas, Publisher.
Page, I. H., et al.: Some observations on the national diet-heart study, Circulation **37:**313, March, 1968.
Raab, W.: Prevention of ischemic heart disease, Springfield, Ill., 1966, Charles C Thomas, Publisher.
Shephard, R. J.: Proceedings of the International Symposium on Physical Activity and Cardiovascular Health, Toronto, Canadian Medical Association Journal **96:** 695, March 25, 1967.
Sprague, H. B.: What I tell my patients about smoking, Modern Concepts of Cardiovascular Disease **33:**881, Oct., 1964.
Wakerlin, G.: Cigarette smoking and the role of the physician, Circulation **29:**651, May, 1964.

T   F

chapter 4
Physical fitness

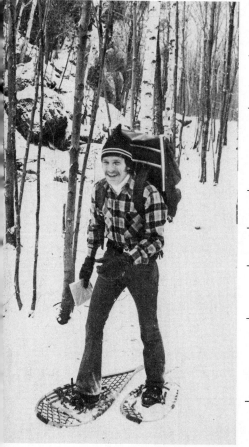

— —   **1.** The increased emphasis on physical fitness during the last 20 years has resulted in a significant improvement in the physical fitness level in this country.

— —   **2.** There is an increased need for man to participate in organized physical activity.

— —   **3.** The incidence in cardiovascular disease is higher in this country than in any other country.

— —   **4.** A large number of people in this country believe that they should exercise more. Most people who do not exercise regularly lack sufficient time to do so.

— —   **5.** Most people in this country exhibit an adequate level of physical fitness.

— —   **6.** The minimal level of physical fitness will be the same for everyone.

— —   **7.** Attaining a maximal level of physical fitness should be a goal for most college students.

— —   **8.** Only factors that relate to the development of health and increase the functional capacity of the body should be classified as physical fitness components.

— —   **9.** The four components of physical fitness are strength, endurance, flexibility, and speed.

— —   **10.** Physical fitness is defined as the ability to perform sports skills correctly.

There is a recognized desire in the United States to improve the physical fitness level of children and adults. The problem was first called to public attention in 1955 by President Dwight D. Eisenhower when he turned his attention to the vital problem of physical fitness. As a former general of the army, he was aware of the inadequate fitness level of young men reporting for military service. Studies made after World War II indicate that nearly 50% of all draft age men had to be rejected or given noncombat jobs because of physical inadequacies.[5]

He also treated with respect and concern the report by Kraus and Hirschland,[4] which indicated that the youth of the United States were inferior to European youth in the performance of six selected tests designed to measure minimal muscular fitness. The results, presented in Fig. 4-1, indicate that in European countries only 8% failed one or more of these tests, whereas 57% failed in the United States. These tests were designed to measure only *minimal* levels of muscular fitness.

As a result, the President's Council on Physical Fitness was established, and following President Eisenhower's example, both President John F. Kennedy and President Lyndon B. Johnson exhibited an extreme interest in the improvement of the physical fitness level of adults and children in this country. President Johnson emphasized that "physical fitness is a matter of fundamental importance to individual well-being and to the progress and security of our nation."[7] President Kennedy referred to physical fitness as "the basis of all other forms of excellence."

Many prominent persons in the field of medicine and other fields have spoken and written about the need for exercise in maintaining an organically sound body from birth through old age. Governors and legislators have called

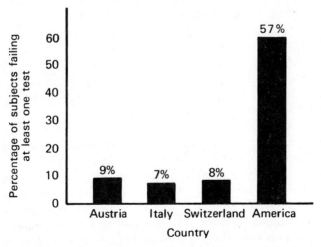

Fig. 4-1. Comparison of European and American children on the Krause-Weber test of minimal muscular fitness. (Adapted from Kraus and Hirschland.[4])

conferences to motivate the people of their states to begin physical fitness programs.

One might ask why the sudden emphasis on physical fitness. One reason is that the tasks of daily life no longer provide sufficient vigorous exercise to develop and maintain "adequate" levels of physical fitness. With increased mechanization there has been a corresponding decrease in the number of tasks that require an expenditure of energy. The result is that many individuals now must rely on various forms of exercise to attain an acceptable level of physical fitness.

There also has been a tremendous increase in "inactive" leisure time activities. As mentioned before, one set of statistics shows that the average American family watches television for 5 hours each day. A second source indicates that school age children spend an average of 21 hours per week watching television.[7] When one considers the number of Americans who spend a large proportion of their weekend in front of the television set watching their favorite professional or college teams participate in athletic contests or actually at the various stadiums as spectators, it would seem obvious why this country has been referred to as a "nation of spectators."

As the following statistics are examined, it is not difficult to see the seriousness and extent of the problem of a low level of physical fitness in this country.

1. Physical fitness tests consistently show American children and adults to be inferior to similar groups from other countries.
2. Over 50% of America's adults are classified as overweight.
3. The incidence of cardiovascular disease in the United States is higher than in any other country in the world.
4. Over 90% of female college freshmen lack sufficient strength to perform one regular pull-up.
5. A large percentage of the American adult population suffer from low back pain as a result of poor muscular development.
6. The American population smoked a record number of cigarettes in 1975.
7. Fifty million American adults do not exercise at all.
8. Forty million additional American adults do not exercise often enough or as vigorously as they need to in order to benefit from this exercise.
9. Lack of physical fitness costs business and industry severely in terms of lost workdays and lowered productivity.

When one considers this information, it would appear that the maintenance of an adequate level of physical fitness is essential for anyone wishing to make the most of himself and of his life and that many advantages result from achieving and maintaining an adequate level of physical fitness. Most Americans are aware of the benefits that can be derived from regular exercise, and many of them intend to exercise more, but for some reason or another they just do not get around to doing this. If a person believes strongly enough in exercise, he will make time available to participate in an activity program on a regular basis. Unfortunately, too few Americans believe strongly enough to do this.

DEFINITION OF PHYSICAL FITNESS

Despite the widespread interest in physical fitness, it is still difficult to define it in a manner that is acceptable to all concerned. The American Association for Health, Physical Education, and Recreation defines fitness as follows:

> Fitness is that state which characterizes the degree to which a person is able to function efficiently. Fitness is an individual matter. It implies the ability of each person to live most effectively within his potentialities. Ability to function depends upon the physical, mental, emotional, social, moral, and spiritual components of fitness, all of which are related to each other and are mutually interdependent.[1]

Clarke defines physical fitness as "the ability to carry out daily tasks with vigor and alertness, without undue fatigue, and with ample energy to enjoy leisure time pursuits and to meet unforeseen emergencies."[1] He further indicates that "physical fitness is the ability to last, to bear up and to persevere under difficult circumstances where an unfit person would give up. It is the opposite to being fatigued from ordinary efforts, to lacking the energy to enter zestfully into life's activities, and to becoming exhausted from unexpected, demanding physical exertion."[2]

Physical fitness is an individual matter and as such has little meaning unless viewed in relation to the specific needs of each individual. The minimal level that is necessary will vary according to the needs of each individual, who must decide for himself whether or not this is sufficient. It is rather unfortunate that many individuals do not realize just how high a level of physical

Table 4-1. Symptoms associated with less than adequate standards of physical fitness*

Symptom	*Check if applicable to you*
1. Yawning at your desk	
2. Drowsy feeling all day	
3. Prone to temper tantrums	
4. Fatigue from minimal exertion	
5. Too tired to pursue leisure activities	
6. Nervous, jittery condition	
7. Difficult to relax	
8. Subject to worries and moods	
9. Irritable disposition toward others	

*Based on data from Cooper, K. H., and Brown, K.: Aerobics, New York, 1968, M. Evans and Company.

fitness is actually necessary. Many persons when asked if they participate regularly in an exercise program indicate that this is not necessary because their level of physical fitness is adequate for their everyday tasks. These, however, are often the same persons who complain of several of the symptoms that are listed in Table 4-1. If several of these symptoms are applicable to you, it is doubtful that you have an adequate level of physical fitness.

As was indicated previously, physical fitness is an individual matter. The amount of activity required by each individual in performing everyday tasks will determine the kind and degree of physical fitness that is necessary. It has been suggested that physical fitness should be considered to exist on a continuum, or scale, ranging from very low levels to maximum levels (Fig. 4-2). Each person has some degree of physical fitness and would thus fit somewhere on this continuum. An individual who is able to meet the demands of each day only with difficulty and who suffers from fatigue and lack of energy would be placed toward the lower end of this scale. According to Johnson et al.:

> The subminimal level of physical fitness is characterized by physical inefficiency and quite often by some degree of emotional instability. He is easily "fatigued," often "edgy" and unable to meet physical or emotional challenges head on with confidence, determination and a reasonable share of success.[3]

It is also possible to consider additional degrees of physical fitness. A person who is able to meet the demands of the day without difficulty and with relative ease would be higher on the scale, toward the maximal level. Somewhere along this scale is a point representing an adequate level of physical fitness. This has been defined as the ability to meet the demands of life with vigor and alertness, without undue fatigue, and to have sufficient energy beyond this to enjoy leisure time activities and meet unexpected emergencies.

There are many points on this scale ranging up to what could be classified as maximal physical fitness. This is a theoretical point, for although it is never actually determined, we know that there is a maximal level for each individual. The highly trained marathon runner, or any highly trained athlete, could be

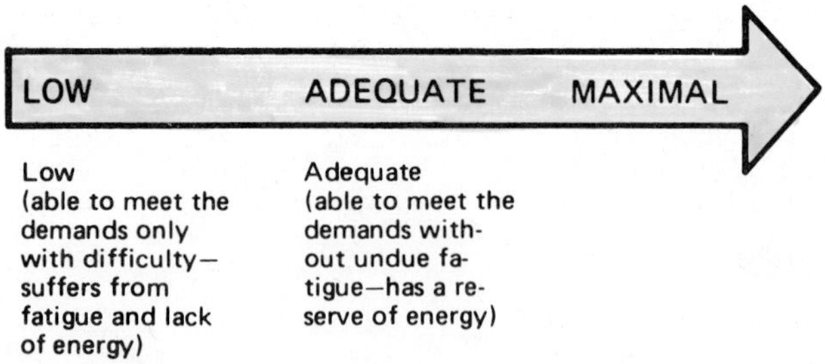

Fig. 4-2. Physical fitness continuum. Each person fits somewhere on this continuum, based on his level of physical fitness. The higher his level of physical fitness, the further he will be toward the maximal level. (Adapted from Johnson, Updyke, Stolberg, and Schafer.[3])

considered as approaching this point. This level, however, is not a required objective for each individual. Each person is fit when his capacities are developed and maintained at a level near his individual capacity for the demands that are most likely to be made on him in the future.[6]

A person can change his position on this scale. If he neglects the needs of the body for physical activity, it will probably result in a shift to the left. A well-designed exercise program that is followed regularly will, in all probability, result in a shift to the right. It is hoped that more people will realize that a minimal physical fitness level may not be sufficient for the ability to meet the demands of tomorrow.[6] An additional level of physical fitness affords the individual an added margin of safety. A greater supply of energy will result in freedom from fatigue and will possibly increase the enjoyment of daily living.

PRESENT STATUS OF PHYSICAL FITNESS IN THIS COUNTRY

Despite the widespread interest in physical fitness during the last 10 years, American boys and girls did not improve their level of physical fitness. Girls have improved slightly in a small number of tests; however, the average fitness scores recorded in 1975 are almost exactly identical to the scores recorded 10 years earlier.[8]

PHYSICAL FITNESS COMPONENTS

To clarify the meaning of physical fitness it becomes necessary to identify and define the contributing components. In the past, several factors associated with the development of skill have erroneously been referred to as physical fitness components. Such factors as speed, balance, agility, power, coordination, and reaction time are factors that are necessary for skillful performance and should be classified as motor ability components, not as physical fitness components.

Only factors that relate to the development of health and increase the functional capacity of the body should be classified as physical fitness components. These are as follows: cardiovascular endurance, muscular endurance, strength, and flexibility. A fifth factor associated closely with physical fitness is weight control. Separate information on each of these components is presented in the following chapters.

REFERENCES

1. Clarke, H. H.: Application of measurement to health and physical education, ed. 4, Englewood Cliffs, N. J., 1967, Prentice-Hall, Inc., p. 14.
2. From Fitness for Youth, Journal of Health, Physical Education, and Recreation **39:** 48, Sept., 1968.
3. Johnson, P. B., Updyke, W. F., Stolberg, D. C., and Schafer, M.: Physical education; a problem-solving approach to health and fitness, New York, 1966, Holt, Rinehart and Winston, Inc., p. 16.
4. Kraus, H., and Hirschland, R.: Physical fitness for children, Research Quarterly **25:**178, May, 1954.

5. Olson, E. C.: Conditioning fundamentals, Columbus, Ohio, 1968, Charles E. Merrill Publishing Company, p. 1.
6. Peebler, J. R.: Controlled exercise for physical fitness, Springfield, Ill., 1962, Charles C Thomas, Publisher, p. 4.
7. President's Council on Physical Fitness: Physical fitness facts, Washington, D.C., 1968, U.S. Government Printing Office, p. 1.
8. President's Council on Physical Fitness and Sports: Newsletter, April, 1976, p. 4.

___ ___ 1. Cardiovascular endurance is the most important component of physical fitness.

___ ___ 2. Endurance is not very important for men who have desk jobs because they do not require very much energy.

___ ___ 3. The main contributing factor to physical work capacity is the strength of the skeletal muscles.

___ ___ 4. The amount of work an individual can perform is largely dependent upon the amount of oxygen the body is capable of processing.

___ ___ 5. The body can store an adequate supply of oxygen.

___ ___ 6. An aerobic task is usually a task that is so vigorous it can be maintained for only a short period of time.

___ ___ 7. A very short task of high intensity is largely dependent upon the supply of energy anaerobically.

___ ___ 8. An activity must produce a maximal heart rate if it is to contribute to the development of cardiovascular endurance.

___ ___ 9. Maximal oxygen intake can be predicted accurately from the results of the 12-minute-run tests.

___ ___ 10. Chinning the bar ten to twelve times daily is one of the best methods for development of cardiovascular endurance.

___ ___ 11. Because of the high level of muscular strength a weight lifter possesses, he will also have a high degree of cardiovascular endurance.

___ ___ 12. The 5-minute step test is just as good as the 12-minute run test for predicting aerobic capacity.

chapter 5

Cardiovascular endurance

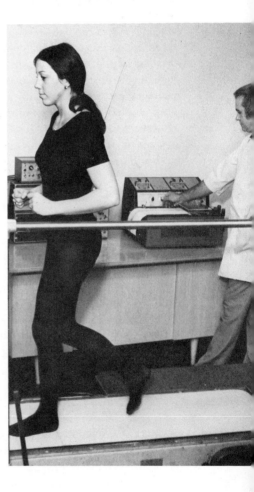

59

Since over 55% of all deaths in the United States are attributable to cardiovascular disease, we should have deep concern for the development of the cardiovascular system. Cardiovascular endurance may be defined as the ability to continue or persist in strenuous tasks involving large muscle groups for long periods of time. In more simple terms it may be defined as the maximal amount of work that an individual can perform over an extended period of time. Large muscle groups should be involved in the work tasks, which should be fairly simple so that the mechanical efficiency is kept relatively constant.

The capacity for heavy prolonged muscular work depends on the body's ability to supply oxygen to the working muscles. The more oxygen the body is able to take in and utilize, the more work the body should be capable of producing. The heart and circulatory and respiratory systems must function efficiently if a high degree of cardiovascular endurance is to be achieved. In recent years this is the one component of physical fitness that has been stressed because of the various health advantages associated with the development of high levels of cardiovascular endurance. It is difficult to determine what advantages are associated with a high level of strength or flexibility, and it has been emphasized that a minimal level of these is adequate for most individuals. However, there are certain benefits that can be derived from attaining above average levels of cardiovascular endurance. These will be discussed in detail in the chapter devoted to exercise and health.

MAXIMAL OXYGEN INTAKE

Just as there is a maximal heart rate that can be attained during exercise, so there is a maximal amount of oxygen the body is able to use. This is referred to as the maximal oxygen intake or aerobic capacity. This measure is recognized by most authorities to be the best measure of a person's cardiovascular fitness.

The amount of oxygen that can be processed by the body is dependent upon the following:

1. *Adequate ventilation.* Air must be moved in and out of the lungs.
2. *Amount of hemoglobin.* This will determine the amount of oxygen that can be carried by the blood.
3. *Cardiac output.* The more blood circulated, the more oxygen that will be available.
4. *Amount of oxygen extracted from the blood.* The ability of the cells to use the oxygen circulated will determine the maximal amount of oxygen that can be used by the body.

The relationship between oxygen consumption and energy expenditure can be summarized as follows:

1. *Each activity requires energy.* Every activity that must be performed by the body requires energy. Even simple activities such as sitting and sleeping require a certain amount of energy.
2. *To produce energy, oxygen is necessary.* Energy is produced by the burning of foodstuffs, but oxygen is the necessary burning agent.

3. *The body can store food, but it cannot store oxygen.* It is necessary for a person to breathe in order to live. If the oxygen supply is discontinued, the body quickly dies, since the oxygen supply in the body will last for only a limited period of time.

When the demands for oxygen increase within the body, as in strenuous exercise, the ability of the body to take in and deliver oxygen to the working musculature will be an important factor in determining how much work can be performed. The more oxygen the circulatory and respiratory systems are able to deliver, the longer the person will be able to exercise before fatigue or exhaustion sets in. As an individual continues running, his performance will deteriorate after a period of time as it becomes difficult for him to continue. The reason is that each person reaches the point at which his body cannot process sufficient oxygen to supply the energy needed to perform the task. Cooper indicates the following when this point is reached:

> . . . each of you should look at what your body is doing in its noble effort to keep you going. Your chest is heaving as the lungs try to bring in more oxygen. Your heart is pounding as it tries to pump more blood which carries the oxygen around your body. The blood is racing through the blood vessels to every extremity as it tries to deliver more oxygen. It's the condition of these systems and others which determines your cardiovascular fitness and it's the improvement of these systems toward which all exercise should be directed.[2]

Aerobic-anaerobic work

The total amount of work of which an individual is capable may be determined by the amount of aerobic work that can be performed, the amount of anaerobic work that can be performed, or a combination of both.

Aerobic work may be defined as work in which the amount of oxygen taken in and used by the body is sufficient to provide the energy necessary for the performance of the task.

Anaerobic work is work in which the amount of oxygen that the body can supply is less than the amount necessary to perform the task. Anaerobic work can be performed *only* for short periods of time, since an "oxygen debt" is incurred, and there is a buildup of lactic acid in the bloodstream.

Balke[1] clearly demonstrates the role of the oxygen debt capacity for the performance of exercises requiring nearly all-out effort for time intervals from 1 to 15 minutes. That a very short effort is accomplished almost entirely anaerobically can readily be seen. The relationship between the two is clearly demonstrated in Fig. 5-1. This graph indicates that during a 1-minute run approximately 60% of the work is performed anaerobically. During a 4-minute run this decreases to approximately 20%, and during an 8-minute task only approximately 10% of the energy is still supplied anaerobically. It can be seen that for work periods exceeding 10 minutes the anaerobic phase becomes less important for the performance of the total work and actually accounts for not more than 5% of the total required amounts of oxygen. This indicates that any task continued for 10 minutes or more gives an adequate estimate

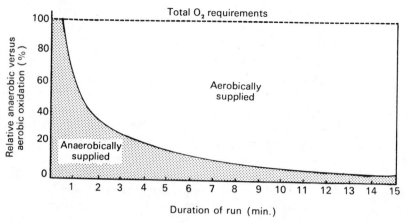

Fig. 5-1. Relative roles of anaerobic and aerobic oxidation for supplying total amounts of oxygen.

of the individual's aerobic capacity if he performs the maximal amount of work during this time period.

DEVELOPMENT OF CARDIOVASCULAR ENDURANCE

Cooper and Brown[2] have indicated that if an activity is to contribute to the development of cardiovascular endurance, it must produce a heart rate in excess of 150 beats per minute and that such improvement begins only after this rate of activity has been sustained for at least 5 minutes. These findings are in agreement with an earlier study by Karvonen.[5] Working with untrained subjects he found that if an activity was to improve the exercise tolerance of the heart, it must produce a heart rate in excess of the value located 60% of the way between the resting and the maximal heart rates. For most of these untrained subjects this critical threshold value was between 140 and 150 beats per minute. To learn which activities are most stressful to the heart and can be used when an overload is necessary for the development of cardiovascular endurance is important. Identifying activities that are less stressful also is important. This information allows the individual to increase the efficiency of his heart by overloading it at times and allowing it to slow down at other times. Activities that satisfy these criteria are considered good activities for the development of cardiovascular endurance. They are usually the continuous activities such as running, swimming, bicycling, basketball, and handball.

A more complete description of the effects of various activities will be presented in Chapter 13.

MEASUREMENT OF CARDIOVASCULAR ENDURANCE

The measurement of maximal oxygen intake is the best measure of an individual's cardiovascular endurance. However, this is not a practical test to administer in terms of either time or equipment, since it involves much time and expensive equipment to administer this test in a controlled laboratory setting.

A reliable estimate of the maximal oxygen consumption may be obtained from the performance during the 12-minute run test. The results of this test correlate very highly (r = +.90) with maximal oxygen intake, and this test is therefore adequate to predict a person's maximal oxygen intake.[3, 4]

12-minute run test

Description of test. During a 12-minute period, each person attempts to run as far as possible and should try to maintain a steady pace throughout. An attempt should be made to increase this speed during the latter part of the performance. The number of laps completed during this time will be counted and recorded, and the actual distance covered in this time period will be calculated.

Results from research clearly show close agreement between the objective criterion of maximal oxygen intake actually obtained in a laboratory situation using the necessary equipment and the estimated values obtained from the results of this field test. One can clearly see that the duration of the running test must be between 10 and 20 minutes to predict the maximal oxygen intake reliably.

Results. The results should be recorded in the spaces provided for them.

Number of laps completed _____

Distance of 1 lap _____ feet
Distance covered = Laps × Distance of 1 lap

= _____ × _____

= _____ feet
To convert to miles, divide by 5,280
Distance covered = Distance covered in feet/5,280

= _____/5,280

= _____ miles (calculate this to 2 decimal places)

Interpretation. The results of this 12-minute field test should be interpreted according to Table 5-1.

Table 5-1. Classification of scores obtained for 12-minute field test

Fitness category	*Men* (distance covered)	*Women* (distance covered)
Very poor	Less than 1.19 miles	Less than 1.01 miles
Poor	1.20-1.23 miles	1.02-1.19 miles
Average	1.24-1.53 miles	1.20-1.27 miles
Good	1.54-1.84 miles	1.28-1.42 miles
Excellent	More than 1.84 miles	More than 1.42 miles

1 ½-mile run test

The 1½-mile run test may be preferred to the 12-minute run test because of the advantage of the ease of administration. The aim of the test is to cover 1½ miles in the shortest time possible. Elapsed time is recorded in minutes and seconds. The results of the 1½-mile run test should be interpreted according to Table 5-2.

Step test

Many different versions of the step test are available for use. Probably the most commonly used is the original 5-minute step test. This test and other variations of it are not as good as the 12-minute run test, but because of practical considerations it is used frequently in the teaching situation.

An accurate measurement of the heart rate is necessary if the results of this test are to be meaningful. Heart rate may be counted most easily by pressing gently with the fingertips on the radial artery that is located on the lateral side of the wrist or on one of the carotid arteries that pass anteriorly in the neck. The place where the pulse can be detected most easily should be used. For the purpose of this evaluation, the pulse will be counted for ½-minute periods and then converted to beats per minute by multiplying the obtained value by 2. Each student will practice counting his heart rate by taking four ½-minute counts while remaining seated. Students should refrain from talking and unnecessary movement during periods when heart rates are being counted, since these activities can influence the results obtained. Results should be recorded in Table 5-3.

Table 5-2. Classification of scores obtained for the 1½ mile run test

Classification	Men (time for 1½ miles)	Women (time for 1½ miles)
Very poor	More than 15 min.	More than 17.30 min.
Poor	14.30-14.59	15.15-17.29
Average	11.45-14.29	14.15-15.14
Good	9.45-11.44	12.45-14.14
Excellent	9.44 or less	12.44 or less

Table 5-3. Heart rate reliability

Trial	Beats per ½ minute		Beats per minute
1	_____	× 2 =	_____
2	_____	× 2 =	_____
3	_____	× 2 =	_____
4	_____	× 2 =	_____

Table 5-4. Scoring for the Harvard step test*

Duration of effort (min)	Total heart beats 1 to 1½ minutes in recovery (score—arbitrary units)											
	40-44	*45-49*	*50-54*	*55-59*	*60-64*	*65-69*	*70-74*	*75-79*	*80-84*	*85-89*	*90-94*	*95-99*
0-½	6	6	5	5	4	4	4	4	3	3	3	3
½-1	19	17	16	14	13	12	11	11	10	9	9	8
1-1½	32	29	26	24	22	20	19	18	17	16	15	14
1½-2	45	41	38	34	31	29	27	25	23	22	21	20
2-2½	58	52	47	43	40	36	34	32	30	28	27	25
2½-3	71	64	58	53	48	45	42	39	37	34	33	31
3-3½	84	75	68	62	57	53	49	46	43	41	39	37
3½-4	97	87	79	72	66	61	57	53	50	47	45	42
4-4½	110	98	89	82	75	70	65	61	57	54	51	48
4½-5	123	110	100	91	84	77	72	68	63	60	57	54
5	129	116	105	96	88	82	76	71	67	63	60	56

Instructions for using this table
1. Find the appropriate line for the time stepping was continued.
2. Find the appropriate column for the pulse count for the 30-second period; do *not* multiply this by 2—it is a 30-second count that is used.
3. Read off the score where this line and column intersect.

*From Consolazio, F., Johnson, R., and Pecora, L.: Physiological measurement of metabolic functions in man. Copyright 1963 and used with permission of McGraw-Hill Book Co.

The step test is based on the premise that for a given submaximal work task the person with a higher level of cardiovascular fitness will have a smaller increase in heart rate and that following the task the heart rate will return to normal much faster than a person's who has a lower level of cardiovascular endurance.

Purpose. The purpose of this test is to obtain immediate knowledge of the level of cardiovascular efficiency.

Method. Students should not perform any type of activity prior to this test, and no warm-up should be allowed. A 20-inch bench should be used for men, whereas a 16-inch bench is recommended for women. Each subject steps up to and down from this bench at the rate of 30 steps per minute. The same foot must start the "step-up" each time, and an erect posture must be assumed. The subject continues the activity for a maximum of 5 minutes or, if unable to continue for 5 minutes, he continues until he is no longer able to maintain the set rate. The heart rate is determined for a $\frac{1}{2}$-minute period, starting exactly 1 minute after completion of the last step, that is, from 1 to $1\frac{1}{2}$ minutes after completion of the task.

Results. The results should be recorded in the spaces provided for them.

Time of stepping _____ seconds

Heart rate _____ beats per $\frac{1}{2}$ minute (1 to $1\frac{1}{2}$ minutes of recovery)

The physical efficiency index (PEI) may be calculated or it may be easily estimated by consulting Table 5-4.

The procedure for calculating the PEI is as follows:

$$PEI = \frac{\text{Time of stepping in seconds} \times 100}{5.5 \times \text{heart rate for } \frac{1}{2} \text{ minute}}$$

$$= \frac{ \times 100}{5.5 \times }$$

$$= \underline{}$$

Interpretation. Results should be interpreted according to Table 5-5.

Table 5-5. Classification of Harvard step test scores*

Score	Cardiovascular classification
Below 55	Very poor
56-64	Poor
65-79	Average
80-89	Good
90 or above	Excellent

*If the lowest row of bleachers is used and these are only 16 inches high, a separate set of standards is presented in the cardiovascular profile chart for men on p. 71.

3-minute shuttle run

This test and the one that follows may give some indication of cardio-vascular endurance even though they are performed for short periods of time.

Description of test. The 3-minute shuttle run is a simple test involving speed, agility, and cardiovascular endurance. Each student runs continuously for 3 minutes back and forth across a badminton court. Each time across the court, the subject touches the outside doubles line with one foot (Fig. 5-2). The aim is to cross the court as many times as possible during the 3-minute period. Each time the subject returns to the starting position, he has scored an additional two laps—one across and one back. The number of single laps completed during the 3-minute time period is counted and recorded.

Results. The results should be recorded in the spaces provided for them.

Number of single laps _____
Distance across court   = 20 feet
Total distance covered = number of single laps × 20 feet

         = _____ × 20 feet

         = _____ feet

Interpretation. Results for the 3-minute shuttle run should be interpreted according to Table 5-6.

1-minute lateral jump test

Description of test. The 1-minute lateral jump test is another simple test involving speed, agility, and cardiovascular endurance. Keeping both feet together, each subject jumps laterally across a line on the floor as many times

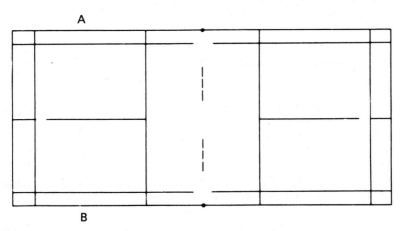

Fig. 5-2. Diagram showing the layout of a badminton court. The two outside lines are identified as A and B. The subject runs across the court and touches one of these lines with his foot. He then turns and runs to the opposite side and touches the other line with his foot. This would constitute the completion of two single laps.

Table 5-6. Classification of scores obtained for the 3-minute shuttle run

Classification	Men (number of single laps)	Women (number of single laps)
Very poor	Less than 65	Less than 53
Poor	65-69	54-58
Average	70-82	59-70
Good	83-87	71-76
Excellent	More than 88	More than 77

Table 5-7. Classification of scores obtained for the 1-minute lateral jump test

Classification	Men (number of single jumps)	Women (number of single jumps)
Very poor	Less than 134	Less than 130
Poor	135-155	131-146
Average	156-180	147-173
Good	181-198	174-183
Excellent	More than 199	More than 184

as possible during a 1-minute period of time. Each time both feet cross the line, this counts as one jump, so that each time the subject returns to the starting position he has an additional two jumps. The aim is to score as many jumps as possible. This can be achieved by jumping close to the line, by bending the knees slightly, and by using the arms to maintain balance.

Results. The results should be recorded in the spaces provided for them.

Number of single jumps completed in 1 minute _____ .

Interpretation. The results of the 1-minute lateral jump test should be interpreted according to Table 5-7.

REFERENCES

1. Balke, B.: A simple field test for the assessment of physical fitness, Washington, D.C., 1963, U. S. Government Printing Office, p. 1.
2. Cooper, K. H., and Brown, K.: Aerobics, New York, 1968, M. Evans and Company, Inc.
3. Doolittle, T. L., et al.: Reliability of the twelve minute run-walk test when employed with adolescent girls, Paper read at the American Association of Health, Physical Education, and Recreation, National Convention, Boston, Mass., April, 1969.
4. Doolittle, T. L., and Bigbee, R.: Twelve minute run-walk: a test of cardiorespiratory fitness of adolescent boys, Research Quarterly **39**:491, Oct., 1968.
5. Karvonen, M. J.: Effects of vigorous exercise on the heart. In Rosenbaum, F. F., and Belknap, E. L., editors: Work and the heart, New York, 1959, Paul B. Hoeber, Inc.

Name _____ Date _____

Day and hour laboratory section meets _____

Laboratory instructor _____

CARDIOVASCULAR EVALUATION
Summary of results

Heart rate reliability

1. _____ beats/min

2. _____ beats/min

3. _____ beats/min

4. _____ beats/min

Step test data

1. Time of stepping _____ seconds
2. Recovery heart rate (1-1½ min of recovery)

 _____ beats/½ min
3. Physical efficiency index _____
4. Cardiovascular classification _____

12-minute field test

1. Number of laps completed _____

2. Distance of one lap _____ feet

3. Total distance covered _____ miles

4. Cardiovascular classification _____

3-minute shuttle run

1. Number of single laps completed _____

2. Distance across court _____

3. Total distance covered _____

4. Cardiovascular classification _____

1-minute lateral jump test

1. Number of single jumps _____

2. Cardiovascular classification _____

1½-mile run

1. Time to complete 1½ miles _____ min _____ sec

2. Cardiovascular classification _____

Name _____ Date _____

Day and hour laboratory section meets _____

Laboratory instructor _____

CARDIOVASCULAR PROFILE CHART FOR MEN

Percentile rank indicates the percentage of students whose score was less than your score. For example, if your physical efficiency index on the Harvard step test was 95, you would have a percentile rank of 70, based on the scores for the 16-inch bench. This would mean that you performed better than 70% of the students who took this test.

Directions

Circle the score closest to that obtained by you on each test. Connect each circle by a line so that comparisons may be made among the four tests.

Percentile rank	Harvard step test (physical efficiency index)		12-minute run (miles)	3-minute shuttle run (number of single laps)	1-minute lateral jump test (number of single jumps)	1½ mile run (min:sec)
	16-inch bench	20-inch bench				
95	115	100	1.92	89	206	9:20
90	108	94	1.84	86	198	9:42
80	101	87	1.74	83	188	10:18
70	95	82	1.67	80	181	10:42
60	90	78	1.62	78	176	11:06
50	86	74	1.56	76	170	11:30
40	82	70	1.50	74	164	12:00
30	77	66	1.45	72	159	12:24
20	71	61	1.38	69	152	13:12
10	64	54	1.26	66	142	14:18
5	57	48	1.20	63	134	15:00
Mean	86.0	74.0	1.56	76.0	170.0	11:30
SD	17.5	11.1	.22	8.0	22.0	1:12

Name _____ Date _____

Day and hour laboratory section meets _____

Laboratory instructor _____

CARDIOVASCULAR PROFILE CHART FOR WOMEN

Percentile rank indicates the percentage of students whose score was less than your score. For example, if your physical efficiency index on the Harvard step test is 66, you have a percentile rank of 30. This means that you performed better than only 30% of the students who took the test.

Directions

Circle the score closest to that obtained by you on each test. Connect each circle by a line so that comparisons may be made among the four tests.

Percentile rank	Harvard step test (physical efficiency index)	12-minute run (miles)	3-minute shuttle run (number of single laps)	1-minute lateral jump test (number of single jumps)	1½ mile run (min:sec)
95	100	1.45	78	186	12:24
90	94	1.39	75	180	12:57
80	87	1.33	72	172	13:30
70	82	1.27	69	167	14:10
60	78	1.23	67	162	14:36
50	74	1.20	65	158	15:00
40	70	1.17	63	154	15:24
30	66	1.13	61	149	15:50
20	61	1.07	58	144	16:48
10	54	1.01	55	136	17:48
5	48	.95	52	130	19:00
Mean	74.0	1.20	65.0	158.0	15:00
SD	11.1	.15	8.0	17.0	1:30

T   F

___ ___   **1.** Overall strength may best be determined by administration of the grip strength test.

___ ___   **2.** Strength of the abdominal muscles can best be measured by the number of bent-leg sit-ups a person can perform in one minute.

___ ___   **3.** Any person who lifts weights regularly will become muscle bound because high resistance exercises limit range of motion.

___ ___   **4.** Strength may best be measured as the maximal amount of force that a muscle group can exert once only.

___ ___   **5.** Isotonic exercises are far superior to isometric exercises for the development of strength.

___ ___   **6.** Strength is really a synonym for muscular endurance.

___ ___   **7.** An isotonic contraction involves exerting muscular force against an immovable object.

___ ___   **8.** Holding a 20-pound weight at arm's length for 10 seconds exemplifies an isometric contraction.

___ ___   **9.** To improve strength one should use light weights and complete as many repetitions as possible.

chapter 6
Strength

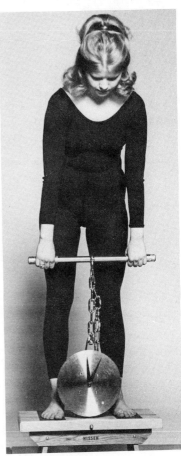

Strength may be defined as the maximal one-effort force that can be exerted against a resistance. For many years this was regarded as the symbol of physical fitness, and many of the physical fitness tests were simply strength tests. A person with well-developed musculature and a good physique was considered to exhibit good physical fitness. However, it should be kept in mind that fitness should not be based on physical appearance but on the functional capacity of the individual to perform work and to supply the necessary energy. The importance attached to the development of strength in increasing one's physical fitness level has declined in recent years. However, it cannot be denied that a minimal level of strength is necessary, for without this it would be impossible to carry out the tasks that are necessary each day. All movement is to a degree dependent on a certain minimal level of strength. A person with poorly developed musculature will find it difficult to maintain an upright posture.

It should also be emphasized that a person who is engaged in hard physical work is going to need a much higher degree of strength than a person who has an office job and spends much of his time sitting behind a desk.

MEASUREMENT OF STRENGTH

Strength is measured correctly by determining the maximal force that a muscle or muscle group can exert once and once only. It is not properly measured by how many times an exercise can be performed or how long an individual can perform a given exercise. These are both measures of muscular endurance and are not measures of strength. For example, it is commonly

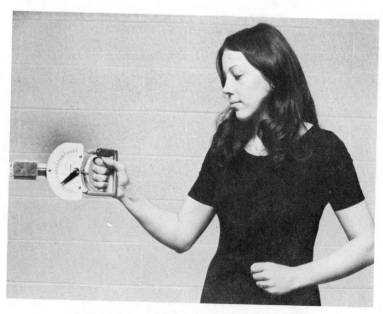

Fig. 6-1. Measurement of grip strength.

thought that the number of push-ups or pull-ups is an adequate measure of strength. These tests actually measure muscular endurance. Grip strength is probably the most commonly used measurement (Fig. 6-1). The subject squeezes the hand dynamometer and exerts a maximal force once and once only as the musculature contracts forcedly. The force exerted is recorded on the dial.

To evaluate strength, many tests must be administered. This is because strength is not a general component but is specific to a particular muscle or group of muscles. Just because one muscle group is well developed does not mean that other groups will be similarly developed. This is known as the principle of specificity. A gymnast, for example, who works on the parallel bars is more likely to have well-developed musculature of the upper body, whereas his muscular development in the legs may be classified as only normal.

DEVELOPMENT OF STRENGTH

Strength may be developed by either isometric or isotonic exercises, or a combination of both.

Isometric training

An *isometric contraction* may be defined as a contraction that occurs when a force is exerted against an immovable object. The length of the muscle does not shorten as a static contraction occurs. An example of this type of contraction would be the measurement of back strength (Fig. 6-2). In this test and other tests like this the subject executes a maximal exertion against an immovable bar, and the force is registered on a gauge.

Isometric training was first made popular in the early 1950s through the research of Hettinger and Mueller,[2] two German physiologists. They showed strength gains from 33% to 181% with isometric exercises performed once daily for 6 seconds per day 5 days a week.

The advantages of isometric training are obvious. A minimal amount of equipment and time is necessary, and large groups of students can participate at the same time. Also these exercises are usually easy to follow, and undue fatigue is avoided.

The major limitation is that isometric exercises can develop strength at only one specific point in the range of motion, whereas with isotonic exercises a *full* range of motion is possible. Also, if a subject cannot see any work being performed, maintaining motivation is often difficult.

The most recent research of Mueller and Rohmert[3] indicates that maximal gains in strength can be achieved by holding a maximal contraction for 5 seconds, five to ten times a day. They also suggest that these contractions be applied at varying points in the range of motion, rather than all at the same angle.

Examples of several isometric exercises that require no equipment follow. These are but a few of the isometric exercises that can be designed to develop the strength and muscular endurance of different muscle groups.

Elbow push. The subject stands with back touching the wall, elbows at

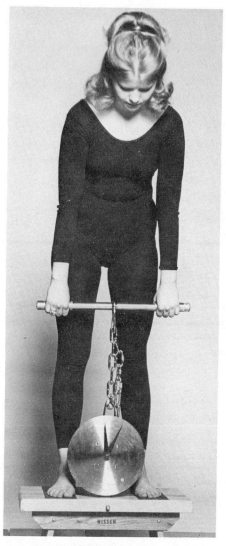

Fig. 6-2. Measurement of back strength—an example of an isometric contraction.

shoulder height and also touching the wall, and forearms flexed and hands beneath the chin with palms down. The elbows are pressed against the wall, as a maximum contraction is held for 5 seconds (Fig. 6-3).

Hand push. The subject stands with the palms together and the elbows raised to shoulder height. The palms are pressed together as hard as possible, and the maximal contraction is then held (Fig. 6-3).

V-sit. For the V-sit exercise the subject sits on the floor, places the hands on the hips, and leans backward until the trunk forms an angle of approximately 45° with the floor. Keeping the legs straight, the feet are raised ap-

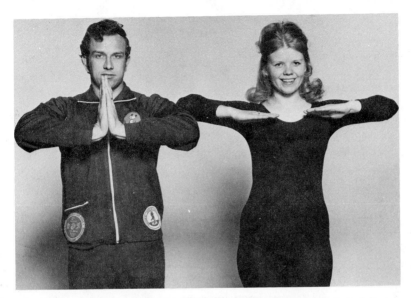

Fig. 6-3. Demonstration of position for the hand push (left) and the elbow push (right). Both of these are examples of isometric exercises.

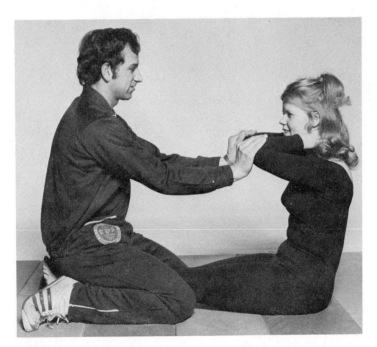

Fig. 6-4. Demonstration of the position to be held for the isometric sit-up.

proximately 12 to 20 inches from the floor as a V position is assumed and then held for a given period of time (Fig. 12-3).

Muscle-maker. The subject flexes the forearm until the elbow joint forms approximately a right angle. The biceps muscle in the front of the upper arm is then contracted maximally, and this contraction is held.

Sit-up. The subject assumes a supine (faceup) position on the floor with the legs out straight in front of him. The upper part of the body is raised off the floor as he sits up, so that the trunk is at a right angle to the legs. A partner straddles the legs and pushes against the chest or elbows (Fig. 6-4). Maximal force is exerted against the force of the partner.

Isotonic training

An *isotonic contraction* occurs when the muscle contracts and shortens and movement takes place. Any time a person lifts a weight through a range of motion (Fig. 6-5), an isotonic contraction takes place. Most common exercises, such as calisthenics and weight lifting, involve isotonic contractions as shortening and lengthening take place. To bring about maximal gains in strength with isotonic methods, few repetitions need to be performed, and the resistance needs to be high. It has been shown that maximal gains in strength occur when the

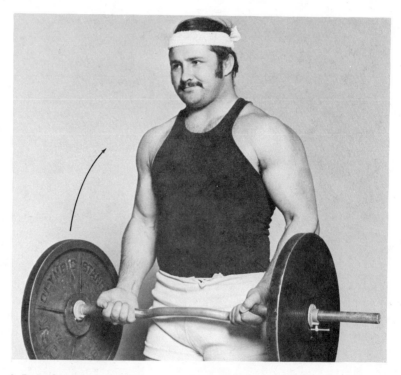

Fig. 6-5. Performance of a two-arm curl—an example of an isotonic contraction as the weight is lifted through a range of movement.

number of repetitions ranges from four to eight and the maximal weight that can be lifted for this number of times is used (Fig. 6-6).

The major advantage of isotonic exercises is that the work can be performed through the full range of motion. Also the individual can see the work being done, which appears to increase the motivation of the participant.

LABORATORY EXPERIENCE
Grip strength

A hand dynamometer is used to measure the force of the hand's muscular contraction. It is placed in the palm of the hand with the dial facing the palm. It is then squeezed as tightly as possible, with the hand and the arm away from the body. It is illegal for the hand or the upper arm to push against any other object or against any part of the body. The score is recorded to the nearest pound in Table 6-1.

To find out how your best score compares with scores from other college students you should circle the score closest to yours on the profile chart at the end of this section.

Table 6-1. Results of grip strength tests (pounds)

	Trial 1	*Trial 2*	*Best*
Dominant hand			
Nondominant hand			

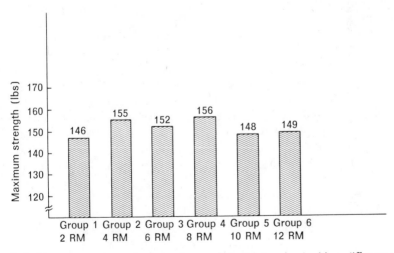

Fig. 6-6. Mean strength results from six groups, each involved with a different training method. (Data from Berger.[1])

Weight lifting exercises for strength or muscular endurance

Two-arm curl. This exercise is designed for the development of the flexors of the forearm. The subject stands with his feet shoulder width apart in an upright position. A barbell is held with the palms-forward grip and the arms extended. With the elbows close to the body, the bar is curled to the shoulder-neck area and returned to the starting position. This constitutes one complete repetition (Fig. 6-7).

Bench press. This exercise is for the development of the chest and shoulders and the extensors of the forearm. The subject lies flat on a bench with the knees bent and the feet flat on the floor. The barbell is held with the palms-forward grip at approximately the width of the shoulders. The bar is then pressed directly upward until the arms are fully extended; then it is returned to the starting position to complete one repetition (Fig. 6-8). The back may not be arched during this exercise but must remain in contact with the bench.

Lateral machine pull-down. This exercise is for the flexors of the forearm, the back, and the upper chest. The subject assumes a kneeling position and the bar is grasped with the palms-forward grip as in Fig. 6-9. The bar is pulled down until it touches the base of the neck and then returned to the starting position to complete one repetition. The body must be kept straight throughout, and no jerking is allowed (Fig. 6-9).

Upright rowing. This exercise is designed for the development of the flexors of the forearm and the shoulders and back. The subject assumes a standing position and grasps the bar with the palms-down grip and the hands approximately 4 inches apart (Fig. 6-10). The bar is then raised until it touches the chin and is then lowered back to the starting position to complete one repetition. The bar must be kept close to the body, and the elbows must remain higher than the hands throughout the lift (Fig. 6-10).

Quadriceps lift. This exercise is designed for the development of the front of the thigh and the extensors of the lower part of the leg. The subject assumes a sitting position with the lower legs at right angles to the thighs and the front of the ankles against the bar (Fig. 6-11). The legs are extended until they are parallel with the floor and then returned to the starting position. The upper body must remain in an upright position throughout (Fig. 6-11).

Leg curl. This exercise is designed for the flexors of the lower part of the leg, mainly the hamstring muscle group. The subject lies face downward with the legs extended and the backs of the heels against the bar (Fig. 6-12). The feet are then lifted upward until they touch the buttocks or are positioned immediately above the buttocks. They are then returned to the starting position (Fig. 6-12).

Curl up. This exercise is for the development of the abdominal muscles. The subject lies flat on the floor with the knees bent, forming an angle of approximately 90° and the feet flat on the floor. The hands are folded over the chest. The subject curls up until the elbows touch the thighs and then returns to the starting position. It is important to avoid jerky movements and to start by bending the head forward slowly (Fig. 6-13).

Text continued on p. 87.

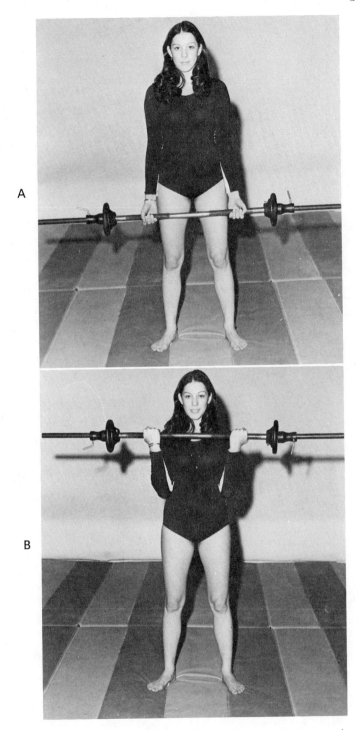

Fig. 6-7. Starting **(A)** and finishing **(B)** positions for two-arm curl exercise.

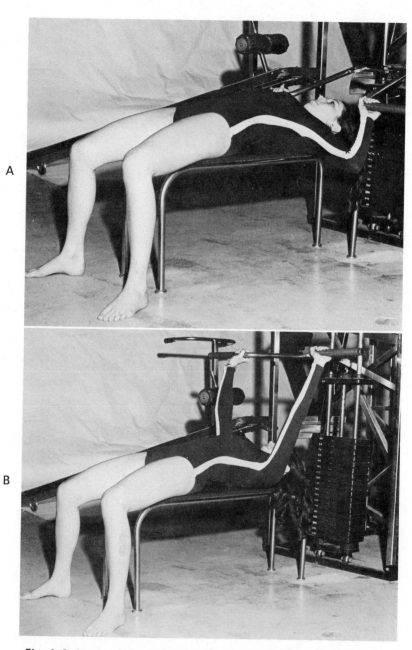

Fig. 6-8. Starting **(A)** and finishing **(B)** positions for bench press exercise.

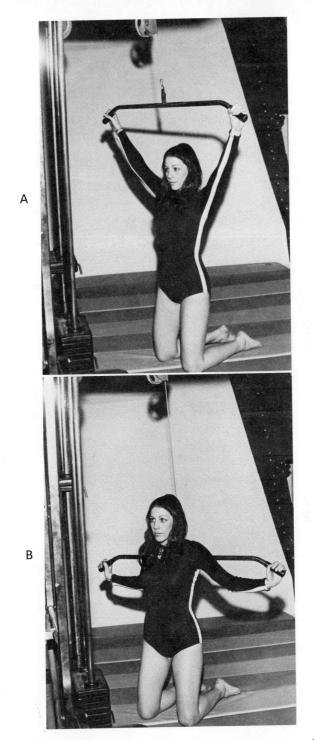

Fig. 6-9. Starting **(A)** and finishing **(B)** positions for lateral machine pull-down exercise.

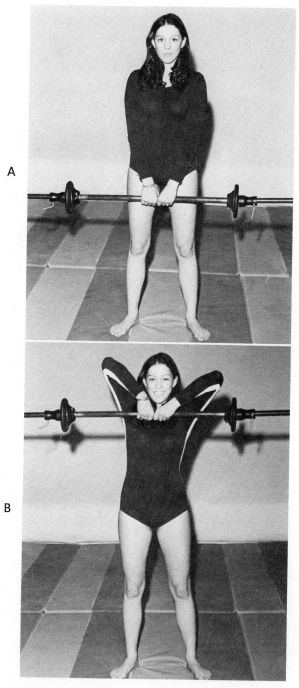

Fig. 6-10. Starting **(A)** and finishing **(B)** positions for upright rowing exercise.

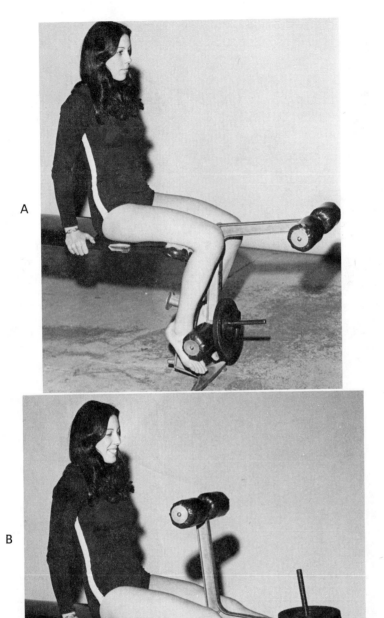

Fig. 6-11. Starting **(A)** and finishing **(B)** positions for quadriceps lift exercise.

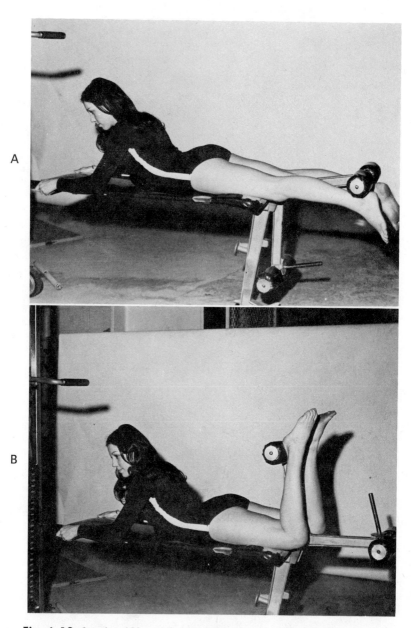

Fig. 6-12. Starting **(A)** and finishing **(B)** positions for the leg curl exercise.

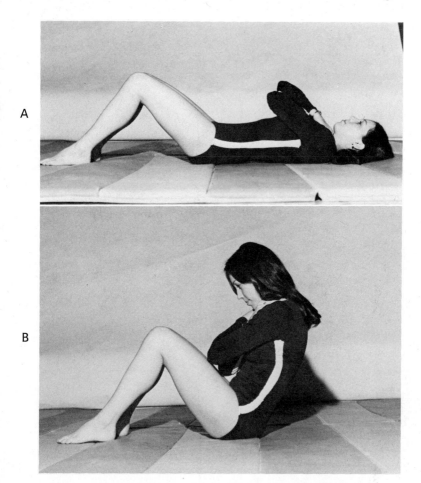

Fig. 6-13. Starting **(A)** and finishing **(B)** positions for the curl-up exercise.

Determination of strength for these tests

To determine the strength for each of these areas, a trial-and-error method must be used to determine the maximal amount of weight that can be lifted once and once only for each of these exercises. This is referred to as one-repetition maximum (1 RM).

REFERENCES

1. Berger, R. A., Optimum repetitions for the development of strength, Research Quarterly **33**:334-338, 1962.
2. Hettinger, T., and Mueller, E. A.: Die Muskelleistung und Muskeltrainerung, Arbeitsphysiologie **15**:111, 1953.
3. Mueller, E. A., and Rohmert, W.: Die Geschwindigkeit der Muselkraftzunahme bei isometrischen Trainierung, Int. Z. Angew. Physiol. **19**:403, 1963.

Name _____ Date _____

Day and hour laboratory section meets _____

Instructor _____

GRIP STRENGTH PROFILE CHART

Percentile rank	Men		Women	
	Dominant hand (pounds)	Nondominant hand (pounds)	Dominant hand (pounds)	Nondominant hand (pounds)
95	159	147	88	83
90	152	140	84	79
80	144	132	79	74
70	138	126	76	71
60	133	121	73	68
50	128	116	70	65
40	123	111	67	62
30	118	106	64	59
20	112	100	61	56
10	104	92	56	51
5	97	85	52	47
Mean	128.0	116.0	70.0	65.0
SD	19.0	19.0	11.0	11.0

Name _____   **Date** _____

Day and hour laboratory section meets _____

Instructor _____

SUMMARY SHEET FOR STRENGTH TESTS

Grip strength

Dominant hand   Trial 1 _____ pounds

Trial 2 _____ pounds   Best score _____ pounds

Nondominant hand   Trial 1 _____ pounds

Trial 2 _____ pounds   Best score _____ pounds

For the following tests, the maximum weight that could be lifted once is recorded.

Two-arm curl   _____ pounds

Bench press   _____ pounds

Lateral machine pull-down   _____ pounds

Upright rowing   _____ pounds

Quad lift   _____ pounds

Leg curl   _____ pounds

Curl up   _____ pounds

T   F

___ ___ **1.** Muscular endurance may be measured by the length of time a particular muscle group can sustain a contraction.

___ ___ **2.** Muscular endurance is the maximal amount of force a muscle or muscle group can exert once only.

___ ___ **3.** Sit-ups should be performed with straight legs for the development of abdominal muscular endurance.

___ ___ **4.** The limiting factors for a muscular endurance task are associated with the heart and circulatory system.

___ ___ **5.** A muscular endurance task performed to exhaustion will result in a near maximal heart rate.

___ ___ **6.** To improve muscular endurance by weight training, keep the number of repetitions constant and increase the resistance each week.

___ ___ **7.** Muscular endurance can be developed by isometric methods in addition to isotonic methods.

chapter 7
Muscular endurance

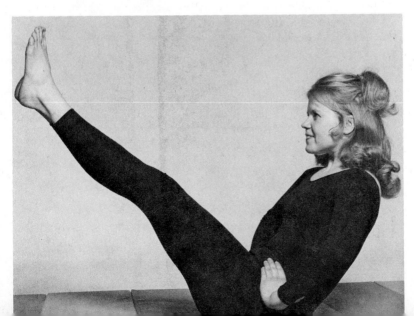

Muscular endurance may be defined as the ability of the muscles to apply force repeatedly or to sustain a contraction for a period of time. Another definition is "the ability to perform work continually involving local muscular effort." For example, if one wishes to measure the endurance of the abdominal muscles, this could be done by determining how many times they can contract within a given time period (bent-leg sit-ups) or how long they can sustain a given contraction (V-sit position).

The longer a muscle can contract without fatigue or the greater the number of repetitions that can be performed before fatigue, the higher the muscular endurance. With this type of work the limiting factor is localized in the muscle group itself, and the circulatory system is usually not taxed to its fullest capacity. Consider, for example, the performance of the simple pull-up. If a student is instructed to do as many pull-ups as possible, a point is reached finally where he is unable to perform any more. He has reached his limit as far as the functional capacity of the muscle group involved is concerned. If the heart rate were monitored throughout, it would show that it is still far from maximal, indicating that the heart and circulatory system are not the limiting factors as far as the task is concerned.

MEASUREMENT OF MUSCULAR ENDURANCE

Muscular endurance is also specific to each of the muscle groups, and because of this many tests are necessary if a complete evaluation of this physical fitness component is to be made. Several of these tests are identified in Table 7-1, followed by a description of the administrative procedures.

Bent-leg sit-up

The bent-leg sit-up is a measure of the muscular endurance of the abdominal muscles. These muscles are very important in maintaining good posture. The subject lies on the back with the fingers interlocked behind the neck. Both feet are placed flat on the floor, and the knees are flexed, forming an angle of approximately 90°. With feet held firmly in place, the subject sits up so that at least one elbow touches one knee (Fig. 7-1). Each elbow *may* touch each knee if the subject desires; however, the most efficient way is to touch one elbow to one knee and to alternate this each time. Each time the subject returns

Table 7-1. Muscular endurance tests

Test	Suggested for men	Suggested for women
Bent-leg sit-up	Yes	Yes
Push-up	Yes	No
Static push-up	Yes	Yes
Pull-up	Yes	No
Flexed-arm hang	No	Yes
Burpee	Yes	Yes
Bench jump	Yes	Yes

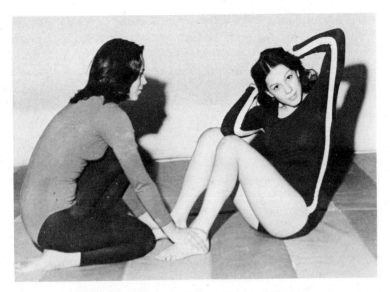

Fig. 7-1. Bent-leg sit-up in test of muscular endurance.

to the starting position, the fingers at the back of the head must come in contact with the floor before the next sit-up is attempted. This process is repeated as many times as possible during a 1-minute time period.

Results. Number of sit-ups in 1 minute _____ .

Push-up (men only)

The push-up is a measure of the endurance of the muscle group concerned with extension of the forearm. The largest muscle of this group is the triceps. The subject assumes a prone position on the floor with hands directly under the shoulder joints, legs straight and together, and toes tucked under so that they are in contact with the floor. The subject then pushes with the arms until they are fully extended. The body is then lowered until the chin or chest touches the floor. At this point there should be a straight line from the head to the toes. All of this movement must be performed by the arms and shoulders and not by any other part of the body. This movement is repeated as many times as possible. There is no time limit to this test, but the push-ups must be performed continuously.

Results. Number of push-ups _____ .

Static push-up

This is a measure of the endurance of the muscle group concerned with the extension of the forearm and is an alternate test to the push-up for men. It is intended for women and is preferred to the modified push-up for women because of the ease of administration and because it is much easier to standardize procedures.

From a straight-arm, front leaning position, with the hands directly under the shoulders, the subject lowers the body until the elbows are flexed to 90° or less. The subject holds this position as long as possible. The test is terminated and the time recorded when any part of the body other than the hands or toes touches the floor or when the body is not maintained in a parallel position to the floor.

Results. Time for static push-up _____ min _____ sec.

Pull-up (men only)

The pull-up is primarily a measure of the endurance of the muscle group responsible for flexion of the forearm. The major muscle of this group is the biceps brachii or, as it is commonly referred to, the biceps. The subject grasps the horizontal bar with both hands, palms facing forward. The "dead hang" position is assumed, with arms fully extended and feet off the ground. The body is raised until the chin is above the top of the bar and is then lowered until the arms are fully extended. The process is repeated until the subject can no longer raise his chin above the bar. The knees may not be raised nor is kicking permitted in an attempt to perform more chinnings.

Results. Number of pull-ups _____ .

Flexed-arm hang (women only)

This test measures the endurance of the flexors of the forearm. Each subject must use the overhand grip with the palms facing forward. The subject then raises the body off the floor to a position where the chin is level with the bar. This position is maintained for as long as possible. Time is stopped when the chin cannot be maintained level with the bar.

Results. Time for flexed arm hang _____ min _____ sec.

Modified pull-up (women only)

In the modified pull-up the bar is adjusted to the height of the sternum, and the feet remain in contact with the floor throughout. The subject grips the bar with the palms forward and slides her feet under the bar until the arms form a right angle with the body. The weight must rest on the heels as the subject attempts to pull up, so that the chin or forehead touches the bar with the body held straight. This is attempted as many times as possible.

Results. Number of modified pull-ups _____.

Burpee

The burpee is a test of muscular endurance involving many large muscle groups. Rapid movements that involve changes in the body position are stressed. The subject stands at attention with feet together and hands at the sides. The squat position is then assumed with the hands placed on the floor adjacent to the feet. The legs are thrust to the rear as the subject assumes the front support position, and at this point the body must be perfectly straight. The feet are brought back to the hands as the squat position is again assumed, and the final step is back to the standing position. As many repetitions as possible are performed in a 1-minute time period.

Results. Number of burpees in 1 minute _____ .

Bench jump

The bench jump is designed to determine the muscular endurance of the muscles of the lower extremity. A 16-inch bench is used, and each subject attempts to jump up to the bench as many times as possible during a 1-minute period. If he is unable to jump he may step up; however, this takes more time. His arms may swing freely, but he is not permitted to push off his thighs when stepping up. One repetition is counted each time both his feet are implanted on the bench and he returns to the floor.

Results. Number of bench jumps in 1 minute _____ .

ALTERNATE MUSCULAR ENDURANCE EVALUATION USING WEIGHTS OR WEIGHT MACHINE

The following method of evaluation of muscular endurance is adapted from Allsen, Harrison, and Vance[1] and is based on the earlier work of DiGennaro.[2] The seven exercises used and the amount of weight used for each person for each exercise are summarized in Table 7-2. It should be noted that these exercises are the same exercises described in detail in the preceding chapter on strength (Chapter 6). The maximum number of repetitions for men is seventeen and for women is fifteen. The resistance in each case is a designated percentage of the body weight of each subject.

Allsen, Harrison, and Vance[1] recommend the following point scale for evaluating each exercise (Table 7-3).

They further suggest that to get an indication of a person's overall muscular endurance the points gained for all seven exercises are added and they should be interpreted according to Table 7-4.

Table 7-2. Muscular endurance tests using weights

Exercise	Body weight	Percent of body weight	Resistance to be used	Repetitions completed	Points earned
Two-arm curl	_____	33⅓	_____	_____	_____
Bench press	_____	66⅔	_____	_____	_____
Lateral machine pull-down	_____	66⅔	_____	_____	_____
Upright rowing	_____	33⅓	_____	_____	_____
Quadriceps lift	_____	66⅔	_____	_____	_____
Leg curl	_____	33⅓	_____	_____	_____
Curl up	_____	14	_____	_____	_____

Table 7-3. Evaluation of muscular endurance tests

| Repetitions | | | Muscular endurance |
Men	Women	Points	category
0-3	0-2	5	Very poor
4	3	7	Poor
5-8	4-7	9	Fair
9-11	8-10	11	Good
12-16	11-14	13	Very good
17	15	15	Excellent

Table 7-4. Overall muscular endurance clarification (total points for all seven tests)

Points	Category
35-48	Very poor
49-62	Poor
63-76	Fair
77-90	Good
91-104	Very good
105	Excellent

REFERENCES

1. Allsen, P., Harrison, J. M., and Vance, B.: Fitness for life: an individualized approach, Dubuque, Iowa, 1975, Wm. C. Brown Company, Publishers.
2. Di Gennaro, J.: Individualized exercise and optimal physical fitness, Philadelphia, 1974, Lea & Febiger.

Name _____ Date _____

Day and hour laboratory section meets _____

Instructor _____

MUSCULAR ENDURANCE PROFILE CHART

Directions

Circle the score closest to the one obtained by you on each test. Connect each circle by a line so that comparisons may be made among the nine tests.

Men

Percentile rank	Bent-leg sit-ups (1 min max)	Push-ups	Static push-up	Pull-ups	Burpee (1 min max)	Bench jump
95	50	53	114	14	40	38
90	47	49	111	12	38	36
80	44	44	106	10	36	34
70	41	41	102	9	35	33
60	39	38	100	8	33	31
50	37	35	97	7	32	30
40	35	32	94	6	31	29
30	33	29	92	5	29	27
20	30	26	88	4	28	26
10	27	21	83	2	26	24
5	24	17	80	0	24	22
Mean	37.0	35.0	97.0	7.0	32.0	29.8
SD	8.0	8.0	11.8	4.0	4.7	4.7

Women

Percentile rank	Bent-leg sit-ups (1 min max)	Static push-up	Flexed-arm hang	Modified pull-ups	Burpee (1 min max)	Bench jump
95	36	38	34	43	30	28
90	33	35	28	40	28	26
80	30	32	19	36	26	24
70	28	30	14	33	24	22
60	26	28	10	30	23	21
50	24	26	8	28	22	20
40	22	24	6	26	21	19
30	20	22	4	23	20	18
20	18	20	2	20	18	16
10	15	17	1	16	16	14
5	12	14	0	13	14	12
Mean	24.0	26.2	8.1	28.0	22.0	20.1
SD	7.4	7.6	2.5	9.4	4.7	4.7

Name _____ Date _____

Day and hour laboratory section meets _____

Instructor _____

SUMMARY SHEET FOR MUSCULAR ENDURANCE TESTS

Men	Number	Percentile
Bent-leg sit-ups		
Push-ups		
Pull-ups		
Burpee		
Static push-ups		
Bench jump		

Women		
Bent-leg sit-ups		
Flexed-arm hang		
Static push-ups		
Modified pull-ups		
Burpee		
Bench jump		

T   F

___ ___   **1.** Flexibility can be defined as the maximal range of movement possible at each joint.

___ ___   **2.** The sit and reach test will give an adequate indication of overall flexibility.

___ ___   **3.** Inactive persons are usually less flexible than active people.

___ ___   **4.** College-age women are much more flexible than college-age men.

___ ___   **5.** Flexibility is specific to each joint.

___ ___   **6.** Possession of adequate flexibility may result in a reduction in the incidence of low back pain.

chapter 8

Flexibility

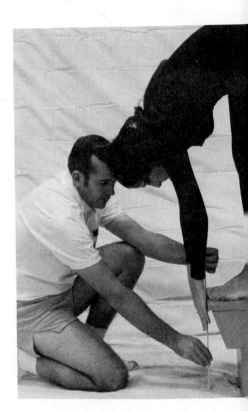

Flexibility may be defined as the functional capacity of the joints to move through a full range of movement. The length of the muscles, ligaments, and tendons largely determines the amount of movement possible at each joint.

It appears as though inactive persons are usually less flexible than persons who are more active. This may be caused by the fact that inactive individuals spend much more time sitting, in which case certain muscle groups are constantly in the flexed position. For example, when a sitting position is assumed, there is usually flexion at the knee joint, at the hip joint, and at the elbow joint. The maintenance of this position for extended periods of time results in these muscles becoming much shorter than they should be. Additional stretching exercises are often necessary if adequate flexibility is to result and if these muscles are to retain their normal length. Without an adequate amount of flexibility one cannot possibly function at his optimal level.

DEVELOPMENT OF FLEXIBILITY

Maintaining adequate flexibility seems to depend on the "amount and intensity of movement of the body parts through complete ranges of motion several times a day." For those whose daily living habits do not result in such movement, it is advisable to participate daily in selected exercises that stress movement of the joints through a full range of motion. Exercises that are performed slowly appear to be more beneficial and less likely to result in injury than exercises that involve bobbing, bouncing, or jerky movements. Isometric exercises can also be used effectively for the development of flexibility.

MEASUREMENT OF FLEXIBILITY

Again it should be stressed that flexibility is not a general component but is specific to each joint. It is therefore not possible to measure flexibility by just one test. Each movement that is possible at each joint must be measured if all aspects of flexibility are to be evaluated.

Leighton[2] has developed an instrument for the measurement of movement at each joint. It is called a Flexometer. Use of this instrument is one of the best methods for the determination of joint flexibility. A number of specific tests have been developed for classroom use when a Flexometer is not available. Three of the more commonly used tests are described below.

Trunk flexion—sit and reach

The degree of trunk flexion will depend on the length of the trunk extensor muscles of the back and also the hamstring muscles. The subject assumes a sitting position with the knees fully extended and the bottom of the feet against the lower board of the bleachers. The hands and arms are stretched forward as far as possible, and this position is held for 3 seconds (Fig. 8-1). A ruler is used to measure the distance in front of or beyond the edge of the bench. Measures in front are negative, whereas measures beyond are positive. This test may also be taken by standing on a bench and reaching down as far as possible (Fig. 8-2).

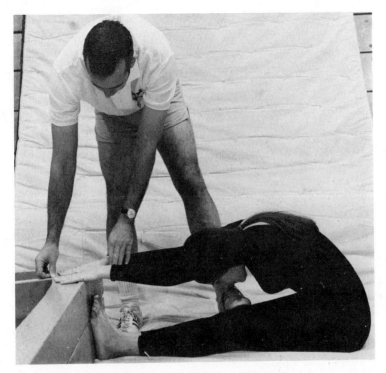

Fig. 8-1. Sit-and-reach test of flexibility.

Results. Trunk flexion—sit and reach _____ inches (be sure to indicate either + or −).

Trunk extension

The trunk extension test is a measure of the range of motion when the back is arched from the prone position. The subject lies facedown on the floor with a partner holding the buttocks and legs down. The fingers are interlocked and the head and shoulders are raised as far as possible from the floor (Fig. 8-3). The distance is measured from floor to chin.

Results. Trunk extension _____ inches.

Shoulder lift

The shoulder lift test measures the range of flexion at the shoulder joint. The subject lies facedown on the floor with his arms parallel and holding a ruler in his hands. The chin and forehead must remain on the floor while the ruler is raised as high as possible with the arms straight. The wrists may not be bent upward in an attempt to achieve a higher score (Fig. 8-4). This position is held for 3 seconds, and the distance from floor to lower edge of the ruler is measured.

Results. Shoulder lift _____ inches.

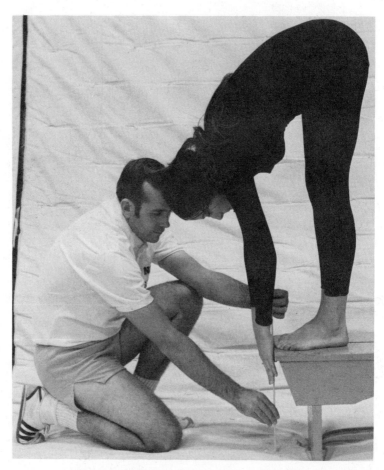

Fig. 8-2. Stand-and-reach test of flexibility.

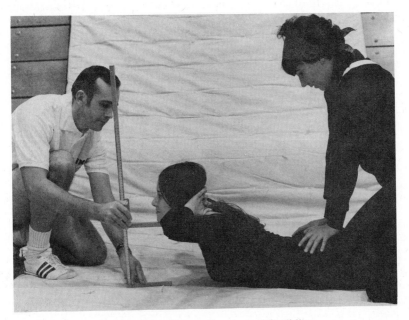

Fig. 8-3. Trunk-extension test of flexibility.

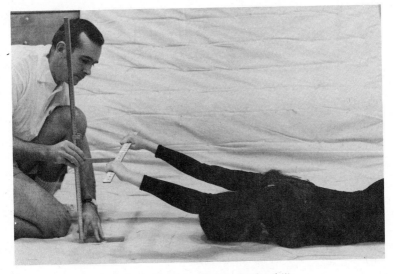

Fig. 8-4. Shoulder-lift test of flexibility.

REFERENCES

1. Falls, H. B., et al.: Foundations of conditioning, New York, 1970, Academic Press, Inc., p. 55.
2. Leighton, J. R.: Instrument and technic for measurement of range of joint motion, Archives of Physical Medicine and Rehabilitation **36:**571, Sept., 1955.

Name _____ Date _____

Day and hour laboratory section meets _____

Instructor _____

FLEXIBILITY PROFILE CHART

Percentile rank	Men			Women		
	Sit and reach (inches)	Trunk extension (inches)	Shoulder lift (inches)	Sit and reach (inches)	Trunk extension (inches)	Shoulder lift (inches)
95	+7.9	24	28	+6.8	22	27
90	+6.9	23	26	+5.9	20	25
80	+5.8	21	24	+4.9	18	22
70	+5.0	20	23	+4.1	17	21
60	+4.3	19	21	+3.6	16	19
50	+3.6	18	20	+3.0	15	18
40	+2.9	17	19	+2.4	14	17
30	+2.5	16	17	+1.9	13	15
20	+1.4	15	16	+0.9	12	14
10	+0.3	13	14	+0.1	10	11
5	−0.7	12	12	−0.8	8	9
Mean	+3.6	18.0	20.0	3.0	15.0	18.0
SD	+2.6	3.8	4.8	2.3	4.1	5.3

Name _____ **Date** _____

Day and hour laboratory section meets _____

Instructor _____

SUMMARY SHEET FOR FLEXIBILITY TESTS

1. Trunk flexion—sit and reach _____ inches

2. Trunk extension _____ inches

3. Shoulder lift _____ inches

What do you know about exercise, diet, and weight control?

T   F

__ __ **1.** An overweight person will also be obese.

__ __ **2.** An obese person has a greatly reduced estimated life span.

__ __ **3.** An overweight person is a person who is 10% or more above his desirable weight.

__ __ **4.** The height/weight charts are the best method available for determination of ideal weight.

__ __ **5.** Skinfold fat measurements are our best means of estimating body fat.

__ __ **6.** Body weight is a dominant factor in determining the energy cost of an activity.

__ __ **7.** Complete starvation for short periods of time is the quickest and best method of weight reduction.

__ __ **8.** Exercise is a very poor weight reduction scheme because one needs to exercise too long to lose a pound of fat.

__ __ **9.** A reduction in calorie intake together with an increase in daily activity is the best means by which a normal person can lose weight.

__ __ **10.** Exercise is of little value in losing weight because if you exercise more you automatically eat more.

__ __ **11.** Vibrating devices are an effective means of reducing body fat from certain areas of the body.

__ __ **12.** Physical effort is essential to neutralize normal caloric intake.

__ __ **13.** Obese individuals are less active than nonobese individuals.

chapter 9
Exercise, diet, and weight control

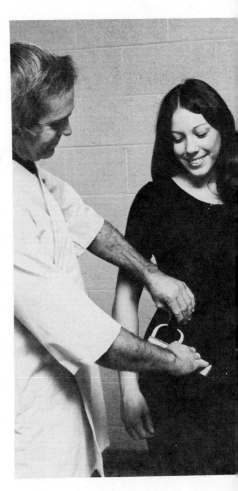

One of the major health problems in the United States today is that of weight control. The American Medical Association has estimated that over 50% of adults in this country can be considered overweight, possibly for one or more of the following causes:

1. Higher standard of living
2. Increased mechanization
3. More lesiure time
4. Less physical activity
5. Insufficient knowledge about weight control
6. Lack of motivation with regard to weight control

Allsen et al. have indicated that "if all the deaths from cancer were eliminated, two years would be added to man's life span and if all the deaths related to obesity were removed, it is estimated that the life span would increase 7 years."[1]

To control weight effectively it is important to study carefully the mechanisms involved. This is most important when one considers the numbers of proposed easy methods available to control weight. Actually, many misconceptions concerning weight control are held by millions of unsuspecting persons.

The purpose of this chapter is to discuss certain common misconceptions pertaining to weight control and present factual information on the importance of exercise and diet.

DIFFERENTIATION BETWEEN AN OBESE AND AN OVERWEIGHT INDIVIDUAL

It is important to differentiate clearly between the terms obese and overweight. An *obese* person is one who has an excessive accumulation of body fat, which raises the question of what the normal or average amount of body fat is. Brozek and Keys[3] indicate that the average percentage of body fat at the age of 20 years is approximately 12% for men and 20% for women. Recent findings from more than 500 students at Northern Michigan University indicate that these are realistic figures for students enrolled at this institution. The average figures obtained were 13% for men and 21% for women.[11] (See Table 9-1.)

Table 9-1. Classification for determination of obesity

Classification	Men (percent)	Women (percent)
Very low	0-8	0-10
Low	9-12	11-15
Acceptable	13-15	16-20
Fat	16-17	21-25
Obese	18+	26+

Mayer[17] suggests that if a quick estimate of obesity is desired, one can measure the amount of fat at the back of the upper arm in the area of the triceps muscle. He suggests that if this measurement is in excess of 15 mm for men or 25 mm for women, these subjects can be considered obese. It should be emphasized that these figures are normal or average figures for college-age men and women. They are not to be considered desirable, for many would agree that they are much higher than they should be.

An *overweight* person is usually considered one who is 10% or more above his desirable weight. Again this raises the question as to what constitutes a desirable weight. Hickman[10] defines the best or desirable weight as "one at which the individual feels well, looks well, is alert and resists fatigue and infection." Originally, simple tables based on a person's height, age, and sex were used to determine the desirable weight. In 1963 the Metropolitan Life Insurance Company[19] introduced a new standard table based on different principles. First, they recognized the undesirability of a continued increase in weight during adulthood past the termination of growth, and second, they realized, at least in theory, that persons vary according to body build. Weight ranges were then presented for three classes of frame size—small, medium, and large. However, to determine in which category each individual was to be classified was apparently left to the subjective judgment of the examiner, since no criteria were presented for classification purposes.

A more recent classification has been prepared by the United States Department of Agriculture. The following method is presented for determination of frame size. Wrist girth is used, and subjects are classified according to Table 9-2.

Tables 9-3 and 9-4 have been modified to indicate the *mean* desirable weight for each of the three classifications for designated heights.

Despite the fact that height-weight tables are used extensively, it should be realized that they do not consider the amount of excess weight that is in the form of fat or the amount that is in the form of muscle.

Most highly trained athletes, particularly football players, would be considered overweight by these standards. However, if these individuals are examined more closely, it can be shown that this excess weight is caused by muscular development and that the percentage of body fat is usually quite low. Garn and Harper[8] concluded that it is not how heavy a person is but

Table 9-2. Frame classification according to wrist girth

Classification	Men (inches)	Women (inches)
Low (small)	5.6-6.7	4.6-5.5
Average (medium)	6.8-7.4	5.6-6.2
High (large)	7.5+	6.3-6.8

Table 9-3. Desirable weights for men 20 to 30 years old (weights listed without clothing according to height without shoes)*

Height (feet, inches)	Weight (pounds)		
	Low	Average	High
5-3	123	129	135
5-4	127	133	139
5-5	131	137	143
5-6	136	142	148
5-7	140	147	154
5-8	144	151	158
5-8	149	155	162
5-10	153	159	166
5-11	156	163	171
6-0	160	167	175
6-1	164	171	180
6-2	168	175	184
6-3	171	178	188

*From U.S. Department of Agriculture: Food and your weight, Washington, D.C., 1973, U.S. Government Printing Office.

Table 9-4. Desirable weights for women 20 to 30 years old (weights listed without clothing according to height without shoes)*

Height (feet, inches)	Weight (pounds)		
	Low	Average	High
5-0	104	109	114
5-1	108	112	117
5-2	111	115	120
5-3	114	118	123
5-4	117	122	127
5-5	120	125	130
5-6	124	129	134
5-7	128	132	137
5-8	131	136	141
5-9	135	140	146
5-10	138	144	150
5-11	142	148	155
6-0	146	152	159

*From U.S. Department of Agriculture: Food and your weight, Washington, D.C., 1973, U.S. Government Printing Office.

how much fat he carries and how much he adds that is important. This would appear to be consistent with the conclusion of Keys and Brozek,[15] who state that "overweight and obesity must be disassociated in order to be understood properly."

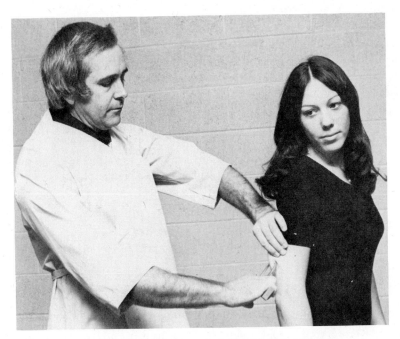

Fig. 9-1. Determination of triceps skinfold thickness.

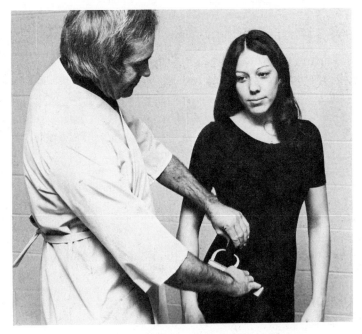

Fig. 9-2. Determination of iliac skinfold thickness.

Determination of percent body fat

By measuring the thickness of various deposits of fat using skinfold calipers, one can estimate closely the body density and percent body fat. Three measurements will be taken for men and two for women. All measurements should be made vertically on the right side of the body (Figs. 9-1 and 9-2).

Results of skinfold tests
Men

   1. Chest skinfold thickness _____ mm.

   2. Abdominal skinfold thickness _____ mm.

   3. Triceps skinfold thickness (arm) _____ mm.

Women

   1. Iliac skinfold thickness _____ mm.

   2. Triceps skinfold thickness _____ mm.

To determine the percent body fat the nomograms presented in Figs. 9-3 (men) and 9-4 (women) must be used.

Results. Percent body fat _____.

Determination of percent overweight using height-weight charts

   1. Record your actual weight to the nearest pound. _____ pounds.
   2. Determine your frame size from your wrist girth.

   Wrist girth _____ inches.

   Frame size (see Table 9-1) _____.

   3. Consult Table 9-3 (men) or 9-4 (women) to determine your desired weight. Desired weight _____.
   4. Determine the difference between the desired weight and your actual weight. Difference _____ pounds.
   5. Divide this difference by your desired weight to determine the percentage you are overweight or underweight. Percentage overweight or underweight (indicate with + or −) _____ %.

Alternate method for determination of desirable weight

The following method, presented by Willoughby,[22] provides a good measure of what the optimal weight should be, taking into account various body-segment widths and diameters.

Six measurements are necessary for both men and women (each is made to the nearest half inch).

   1. *Shoulder width* (use wooden calipers and measure from the tip of the acromial process to the tip of the acromial process on the other side) (Fig. 9-5).

   Shoulder width = _____ inches.

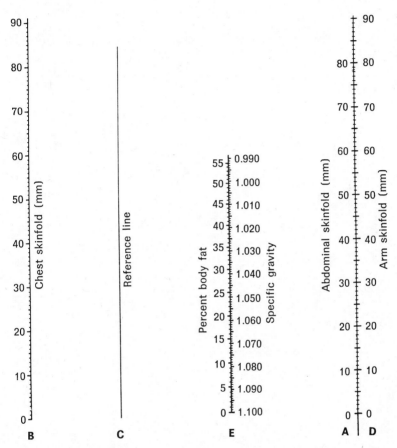

Fig. 9-3. Example of nomogram for conversion of skinfold thickness to specific gravity and percent fat in young men. Given: Abdominal skinfold 10 mm, chest skinfold 15 mm, and arm skinfold 20 mm. (1) With straight edge align abdominal value (10 mm) in column A with chest value (15 mm) in column B. (2) Place pin at point where straight edge crosses reference line C. (3) Pivot straight edge on pin to arm skinfold value (20 mm) in column D. (4) Read specific gravity (1.070) and percent body fat (14%) where straight edge crosses column E. Specific gravity $= 1.1017 - 0.000282A - 0.000736B - 0.000883D$. (Brozek, J., and Keys, A.: British Journal of Nutrition **5**:194, 1951. Sample: 116 men, 18 to 26 years old.) Percent body fat $= 100 (5.548/sp\ g - 5.044)$. (Rathbun, E. N., and Pace, N.: Journal of Biology and Chemistry **158**:667, 1945. Theoretically derived formula.) (Modified from Consolazio, C. F., et al.: Physiological measurements of metabolic functions in man, New York, 1963, McGraw-Hill Book Company. Used by permission of McGraw-Hill Book Company.)

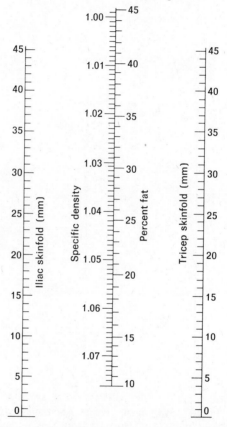

Nomogram for conversion of skinfold thickness of specific
gravity and percent fat in young women

Fig. 9-4. Nomogram for conversion of skinfold thickness to percent body fat for use
with young women. (From Corbin, C., et al.: Concepts in physical education, Dubuque,
Iowa, 1970. Used by permission of Wm. C. Brown Company, Publishers.)

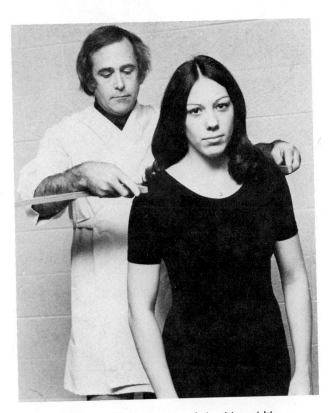

Fig. 9-5. Determination of shoulder width.

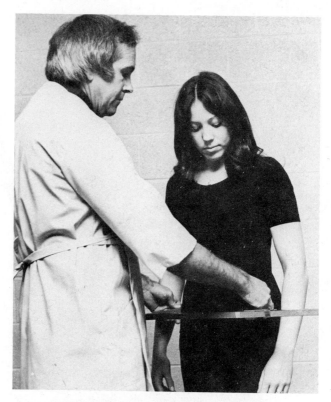

Fig. 9-6. Determination of iliac width.

2. *Iliac width* (use wooden calipers and measure from iliac crest to iliac crest; Fig. 9-6).

Iliac width = _____ inches.

3. *Hip width* (use wooden calipers and measure from the most lateral point on each side of the upper part of the femur; Fig. 9-7).

Hip width = _____ inches.

4. *Wrist girth* (use tape measure and include the *bony knob*).

Wrist girth = _____ inches.

5. *Knee girth* (use tape measure and measure at the middle of the patella).

Knee girth = _____ inches.

6. *Ankle girth* (use tape measure and measure at the *smallest* point—do not include the bony knob).

Ankle girth = _____ inches.

The following calculations are necessary:

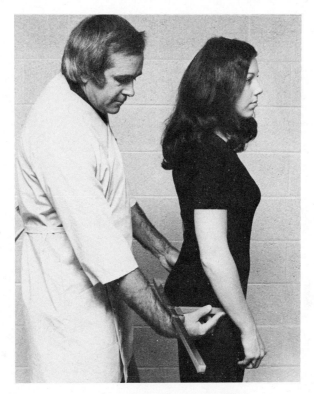

Fig. 9-7. Determination of hip width.

For women

0.59 × Shoulder width = _____

0.75 × Iliac width   = _____

1.33 × Hip width   = _____

2.70 × Wrist girth   = _____

1.77 × Knee girth   = _____

3.00 × Ankle girth   = _____

Total   = _____

Corrected ankle girth = Total/12

                      = _____

For men

0.55 × Shoulder width = _____

0.78 × Iliac width   = _____

1.36 × Hip width   = _____

2.28 × Wrist girth   = _____

1.78 × Knee girth   = _____

3.00 × Ankle girth   = _____

Total   = _____

Corrected ankle girth = Total/12

                      = _____

The optimal weight per inch of height is now determined by consulting Table 9-5 for the figure that corresponds to your corrected ankle girth.

Table 9-5. Desirable weight per inch of height for men and women

Corrected ankle girth	Desirable body weight per inch of height	
	Women	Men
7.0	1.41	—
7.1	1.45	—
7.2	1.50	—
7.3	1.54	—
7.4	1.58	1.72
7.5	1.62	1.77
7.6	1.67	1.81
7.7	1.71	1.86
7.8	1.75	1.91
7.9	1.80	1.96
8.0	1.85	2.01
8.1	1.89	2.06
8.2	1.94	2.11
8.3	1.99	2.16
8.4	2.04	2.21
8.5	2.08	2.27
8.6	2.13	2.32
8.7	2.18	2.37
8.8	2.23	2.43
8.9	2.28	2.49
9.0	2.34	2.54
9.1	2.39	2.60
9.2	2.44	2.66
9.3	2.50	2.71
9.4	2.54	2.77
9.5	—	2.83
9.6	—	2.89
9.7	—	2.95
9.8	—	3.01
9.9	—	3.07
10.0	—	3.14

Multiply your height (inches) by the figure obtained from Table 9-5 to find your desirable weight.

Desirable weight = _____ pounds.

FOODS REQUIRED BY THE BODY

The three basic foodstuffs are fats, proteins, and carbohydrates. During the process of digestion each of these is broken into its simplest form and used as a source of energy or for the production of new tissue.

Protein. Protein is needed primarily to build, repair, and regulate the function of the body's cells. It is found mainly in meat, fish, poultry, eggs, milk, cheese, and bread. Proteins constitute approximately 15% of the average American diet.

Carbohydrate. Carbohydrate is the major source of energy for the body. Carbohydrates make up approximately 45% of the typical American diet and often are referred to as starches and sugars. Foods that are high in carbohydrate content are fruits, bread, milk, and potatoes.

Fat. Fat is a secondary source of energy and makes up about 40% of the average American diet. It is found primarily in butter, margarine, oils, meat, whole milk, chocolate, and nuts. Moderate deposits of fat in the body tissues serve as a reserve fuel supply, and some deposits are necessary for the support and protection of certain vital organs. However, excessive deposits may result in added stress on the heart and joints and can result in decreased functioning of the body.

ENERGY

Energy may be defined as the capacity to perform work. Actually, there are two types of energy: (1) potential—stored energy—and (2) kinetic—active energy. Just as the automobile can convert gasoline to power, so the human body converts potential energy from food into kinetic energy in the form of heat and work.

The Calorie

The common unit of measurement for measuring energy is the Calorie, or, as it is commonly known, the kilocalorie. One kilocalorie is the amount of heat that is necessary to raise 1 kg of water 1° Celsius. It can be used to express the potential energy of food and the amount of energy used by the body in performing various activities.

Caloric intake

The caloric content of the food ingested can be measured. To determine the number of Calories in any food, the food is dehydrated and burned in a special piece of equipment, called a calorimeter. When the food is burned, the increase in temperature is measured, and thus the caloric content of the food is determined. The caloric equivalent for each of the three basic foods is presented in Table 9-6.

It can be seen that if the total amount of carbohydrate, fat, and protein is known, caloric equivalents for various foods can be determined. These have

Table 9-6. Energy available from the three basic types of food

Type of food	Calories/gram
Carbohydrates	4.0
Fats	9.0
Proteins	4.0

Table 9-7. Caloric values for certain selected foods

Food	Serving	Calories
Apple	1 small	75
Apple pie	⅙	275
Applesauce (can)	½ cup	100
Apricots	5 medium	100
Asparagus	12 stalks	25
Bacon (fried)	3 strips	100
Banana	1	100
Banana split	1	450
Beef Stroganoff	average	350
Blueberry muffin	average	150
Bologna	2 ounces	125
Bouillon	1 cup	25
Bread	1 slice	65
Butter	1 pat	50
Cantaloupe	½	50
Cauliflower	1 cup	30
Cheese (American)	1 slice	100
Cheesecake	1 average	350
Chewing gum	1 stick	6
Chicken (baked)	average	200
Chili	½ cup	175
Chocolate bar	average	100
Chocolate cake	1 average	250
Cinnamon roll	average	100
Clams	12 medium	100
Cocoa (with milk)	1 cup	235
Coffee (black)	1 cup	0
Coffee (with cream)	1 cup	30
Coffee (with cream and sugar)	1 cup	65
Coleslaw	6 ounces	20
Corn (fresh frozen)	1 cup	140
Cornflakes	1 cup	100
Corned beef	4 ounces	250
Cottage cheese	1 cup	215
Crackers, graham	3 medium	75
Crackers, soda	6	100
Cream cheese	1 tablespoon	50
Cupcakes (iced)	1 small	150
Dressing (Italian)	1 tablespoon	50
Dressing (Thousand Island)	1 tablespoon	100
Egg (boiled)	1	75
Egg (scrambled)	1	150
Fish (haddock)	average	180
Fish (tuna)	½ cup	250
Frankfurter	1 average	125

Table 9-7. Caloric values for certain selected foods—cont'd

Food	Serving	Calories
Frankfurter roll	1	125
French toast	1 slice	125
Fudge	1-inch square	110
Ginger ale	6 ounces	75
Grapefruit	½ small	50
Ham (baked)	average	350
Hamburger (broiled)	2 ounces	200
Hot fudge sundae	2 scoops	400
Ice cream (vanilla)	average	150
Ice cream soda	1	350
Jam (strawberry)	1 tablespoon	50
Jello	average	100
Lamb chop	1-inch thick	250
Lemon meringue pie	1 piece	350
Lettuce	¼ head	10
Lobster tail	4 ounces	100
Macaroni and cheese	½ cup	225
Martini	1	125
Meat loaf	average	225
Milk	¾ cup	125
Milk (skimmed)	1 cup	85
Muffins	1 average	125
Nuts (Brazil)	2 average	50
Olives	6 small	50
Omelet (cheese)	2 eggs	200
Onion (fried)	1	150
Onion (raw)	1 large	50
Onion soup (French)	8-ounce cup	150
Orange	1 medium	75
Orange juice (can)	4 ounces	70
Pancakes	1 4½-inch diameter	100
Peaches	1 medium	50
Peanut butter	1 tablespoon	100
Pickles (dill)	1 large	15
Pickles (sweet)	1 small	25
Pizza with sausage	⅙ (12-inch diameter)	250
Pork chop	1 medium	225
Potato (baked)	1 medium	125
Potato (mashed)	1	180
Potato (hashed brown)	1 medium	225
Potato (french fried)	6	100
Potato chips	½ cup	100
Pretzels	6	100
Pudding (chocolate)	½ cup	250
Ravioli	1	75

Continued.

Table 9-7. Caloric values for certain selected foods—cont'd

Food	Serving	Calories
Roast beef	6 ounces	75
Salt	⅛ teaspoon	0
Soup (chicken noodle)	1 cup	125
Sour cream	¼ cup	200
Spaghetti with meat sauce	1 serving	375
Spare ribs	6	250
Steak (porterhouse)	average	400
Steak (T-bone)	average	200
Tomato (fresh)	1 medium	25
Tomato juice	1 cup	50
Turkey	average	175
Waffle	1	225
Water	1 cup	0
Wheat (puffed)	1 ounce	105
Wine (white)	wine glass	135
Yogurt	1 cup	165

been calculated, and the values for certain selected foods are presented in Table 9-7. A more detailed table may be found in most nutrition books.

Energy expenditure

The energy expenditure of each activity may be calculated by measuring the amount of oxygen used in performing the activity. There is a direct relationship between energy expenditure and oxygen consumption because oxygen is used to burn food in producing the necessary energy. It takes approximately 1 liter of oxygen to burn 5 Calories of food. The amount of oxygen used by the body is obviously an important measurement. For example, if a person exercises so that he uses 4 liters of oxygen per minute, for each minute that he continues to exercise he will use 4 × 5, or 20, Calories—equivalent to 1,200 Calories for each hour that he exercises. This is a very fast rate of work and would correspond to marathon running at a rate of approximately 12 miles per hour. It is therefore possible to have a subject perform an activity for a given time and to measure the amount of oxygen that is used. This in turn can then be converted to the number of Calories used in performing the task.

The energy expenditure for different tasks will vary according to the person's skill level, body weight, and other factors. However, it is possible to obtain a good approximation of a person's energy expenditure by consulting tables prepared from actual measurements. The energy expenditure figures for certain selected activities are given in Table 9-8.

It should be stressed that these are average figures and will vary according to skill level. The difference attributable to weight can be determined by taking the Calories per minute per pound and multiplying by the number of pounds that the person weighs and the number of minutes that the activity is per-

Table 9-8. Energy expenditure for certain selected physical activities*

Activity	Cal/min/lb	Activity	Cal/min/lb
Archery	.034	Running	
Badminton		5.5 mph	.071
Moderate	.038	6.0 mph	.080
Vigorous	.065	7.0 mph	.090
Bowling	.030	9.0 mph	.100
Baseball	.030	10.0 mph	.115
Basketball		12.0 mph	.130
Half court	.028	Sailing	.020
Moderate	.045	Soccer	.063
Competitive	.066	Squash	.070
Bicycling		Snowshoeing (2.5 mph)	.067
Slow (5.5 mph)	.025	Swimming	
Moderate (10 mph)	.050	Crawl stroke at 1 mph	.045
Fast (13 mph)	.071	(rate 25 yd in 51 sec)	
Canoeing		Crawl stroke at 1.6 mph	.076
Slow (2.5 mph)	.023	(rate 25 yd in 31 sec)	
Fast (4.0 mph)	.047	Crawl stroke at 2.2 mph	.176
Calisthenics	.033	(rate 25 yd in 23 sec)	
Dancing		Recreational	.038
Moderate	.030	Skiing	
Vigorous	.045	Downhill	.060
Fishing	.016	Level (5 mph)	.078
Football	.060	Skating	
Golf	.036	Moderate	.040
Gymnastics		Vigorous	.065
Light	.022	Tennis	.040
Heavy	.056	Table tennis	.030
Handball	.065	Volleyball	.030
Hiking	.065	Walking	
Hill climbing	.060	2 mph	.020
Judo and karate	.087	3.5 mph	.031
Paddleball	.066	4.5 mph	.082
Pool	.025	In 12-18 inches snow	.082
		Water skiing	.053
		Wrestling	.053

*Values are adapted from a number of different sources, including references 18, 19, 20, and 21.

formed. For example, if a person weighing 200 pounds ran at 5 miles per hour for 30 minutes, he would use 0.050 × 30 × 200, or 300 Calories for the half hour.

Energy balance

Regardless of whether a person tries to control weight by diet or by exercise, it is the balance between food intake and energy expenditure that will determine whether the program will be successful or not.

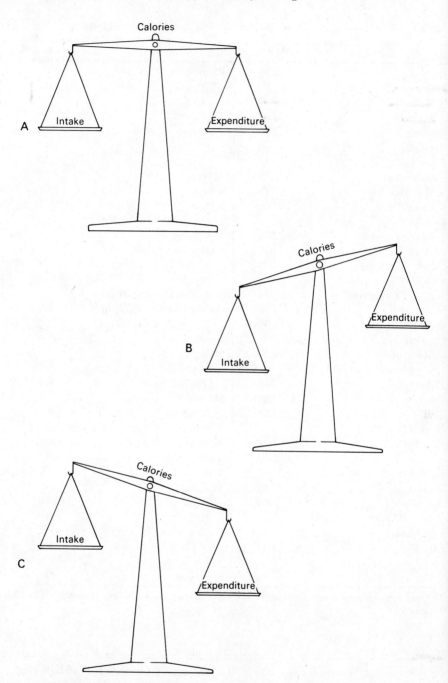

Fig. 9-8. A, Neutral energy balance, in which caloric intake and caloric expenditure are balanced. **B,** Positive energy balance, in which the caloric intake is greater than the caloric expenditure. **C,** Negative energy balance, in which the caloric expenditure is greater than the caloric intake.

A neutral energy balance exists when the caloric intake is equal to the caloric expenditure (Fig. 9-8, *A*). Under these conditions the body weight should remain constant and should neither increase nor decrease by any appreciable amount.

A positive energy balance exists when the caloric intake is greater than the caloric expenditure (Fig. 9-8, *B*). The excess food is stored in the form of fat, and the body weight will increase.

In a negative energy balance situation, the exact opposite is true. The number of Calories used will be greater than the number of Calories consumed (Fig. 9-4, *C*). The extra energy is supplied by the burning of fat, and the body fat and weight will be reduced.

Caloric equivalent of one pound of fat

A few simple calculations make it possible to determine how many Calories are the equivalent of 1 pound of fat. The following information is known:

$$1 \text{ gram of fat} = 9 \text{ Calories}$$
$$1 \text{ pound of fat} = 453 \text{ g}$$

Thus the caloric equivalent of 1 pound of fat is 453 × 9, or 4,077 Calories.

If a person takes in 4,000 Calories a day and uses only 3,000, then each day he takes in approximately 1,000 Calories more than he uses. Obviously, for each four days that this situation exists he will accumulate an excess of 4,000 Calories, which is approximately equivalent to 1 pound of fat.

Table 9-9. Energy expenditure for everyday tasks*

Everyday tasks	Cal/min/lb	Everyday tasks	Cal/min/lb
Sleeping	.008	Standing, light activity	.016
Lying quietly	.009	House painting	.023
Sitting eating	.011	Sweeping floors	.024
Mental work, seated	.011	Dressing and showering	.024
Sitting	.011	Carpenter work	.025
Standing	.012	Making bed	.027
Conversing	.012	Cleaning windows	.028
Sitting writing	.012	Ironing	.028
Washing dishes	.012	Farming and planting	.031
Cooking	.013	Gardening	.032
Lecturing	.014	Pick and shovel work	.043
Driving a car	.015	Shoveling sand	.044
Office work	.016	Chopping wood	.049
Light housework	.016		

*Values are adapted from a number of different sources including references, 18, 19, 20, and 21.

Determination of caloric intake

For an individual to obtain a good indication of his caloric intake, he should select a typical weekday and a typical day of the weekend. He should record carefully everything consumed on these days and convert that to Calories by consulting a table of caloric food values. For a more accurate indication of caloric intake, determinations should be made for several such days. The data obtained should be presented on p. 135. If a more accurate indication is desired, both the caloric intake and caloric expenditure should be kept over several days.

Determination of caloric expenditure

For an individual to obtain a good indication of his caloric expenditure, he should estimate the time spent at different activities for the same two days used for the caloric intake. The energy expenditure listing in Table 9-9 should be consulted to determine the number of Calories involved. These data should be recorded on p. 136.

The obtained results should be summarized in Table 9-10 and determination made, on this basis, of how the weight should be adjusted.

WEIGHT CONTROL
Exercise as a means of controlling weight

Many persons who are genuinely concerned with losing excess weight have concentrated only on counting the number of Calories in their diets and have completely neglected the role that increased activity can play. For those who are overweight, increasing the amount of physical activity can be just as important as decreasing the food intake. A sensible approach involves a dietary restriction with a progressive buildup of exercise. If a person simply reduces his intake by 400 Calories per day, it will take him ten days to lose a pound of fat should his activity level remain constant. However, if he increases his ac-

Table 9-10. Determination of energy balance

	Day 1	Day 2
Total Calories extended		
Total caloric intake		
Difference		
Energy balance (positive or negative)		
Estimated number of pounds you should lose/gain during one year*		

*One pound of fat = 4,000 Calories.

tivity level by playing an hour of tennis per day or walking an additional hour per day, then it may take him just five days to lose the pound of fat.

Several studies have indicated that lack of exercise is the most important cause of the "creeping" obesity found in modern mechanized society. Rony,[21] for example, suggests that laziness, or a decreased tendency toward muscular activity, is a primary characteristic of obese children. He was able to show that they avoided unnecessary activity, outdoor play, and athletics. In a similar study, Bronstein et al.[2] found that most of the thirty-five obese children who were studied spent most of their leisure time in sedentary activities. Green[9] studied more than 200 overweight adult patients in whom the beginning of obesity could be traced directly to a sudden decrease in activity.

When one considers that few occupations now require vigorous physical activity, it is understandable that a large percentage of the adult population is considered overweight. For although there is more time available for recreation, few people use this time in activities that give them exercise.

Misconceptions concerning weight control

Until recent years the role of exercise in weight control programs has been minimized. The reason for this appears to be that many persons lack sufficient information concerning the relationship between exercise and weight control. Also two basic *misconceptions* relating to the role of exercise in weight control have been widely held. Mayer summarizes these as follows:

1. Exercise requires relatively little caloric expenditure and, therefore, increased physical activity hardly changes the caloric balance.
2. An increase in physical activity is always automatically followed by an increase in appetite and food intake and may, therefore, actually impair the success of the weight control program.[16]

Scientific evidence relating to these statements clearly shows that both of them are false.[14]

Energy expenditure in exercise

The average adult man will use from 2,400 to 4,500 Calories a day, depending on the level of activity. Persons who are very active, such as laborers and athletes, may require as many as 6,000 Calories per day—a fact that has been known for many years. Johnson[14] has shown that when a group of university students increased their caloric expenditure from 3,000 to 6,000 Calories per day, they were able to maintain a constant weight by increasing the amount of exercise in which they participated each day.

It was shown previously that 1 pound of fat is equivalent to approximately 4,000 Calories. The caloric expenditure for certain tasks also was presented. It is possible therefore to calculate the number of hours that must be spent participating in an activity to lose 1 pound of fat. These figures are presented in Table 9-11 for certain selected activities.

This information suggests that losing weight through exercise would be dif-

Table 9-11. Caloric expenditure and weight control for certain activities, for a 170-pound man

Activity	Cal/hr	Hours to lose 1 pound of fat
Walking	337	11.8
Basketball	479	8.4
Volleyball	235	17.0
Golf	367	10.9
Tennis	469	8.5
Wrestling	950	4.2

ficult. For example, one would have to play volleyball for 17 hours to lose 1 pound of fat. This is equivalent to 10.9 hours of golf or 8.5 hours of tennis. The fact that has been overlooked, however, is that the activity does not have to be performed continuously. One must look at the "long haul" concept of weight control. If a person plays tennis for 1 hour a day, 4 days a week, over a period of a year, this will account for approximately 25 pounds. This emphasizes one point: for exercise to be beneficial it must be performed regularly. Another point is important. If a person walked an extra mile a day instead of riding, this would account for a loss of almost 30 pounds over a period of a year, provided his caloric intake remained constant. This is really not an impractical amount of time to spend, and if it is desirable to lose weight faster or to lose more weight, it simply becomes necessary to increase the amount of activity.

Food intake and exercise

The claim that an increase in physical activity always causes an increase in appetite and food intake that equals or is greater in energy value than the energy cost of the exercise also is false. Laboratory tests using rats have shown that when the amount of exercise performed is moderate, from 20 minutes to 1 hour, the food intake does not increase—in fact, it actually shows a decrease. These results are presented in Fig. 9-9. Not only was there a decrease in the daily caloric intake, but there was also a decrease in body weight. With long periods of sustained activity the food intake did increase, but the weight remained constant at this optimal level, since the extra activity balanced out the extra caloric intake.

Mayer[17] also was able to obtain similar results working with adults. This study was conducted in 1954 in India, where it was possible to control adequately many relevant factors. The results of this study are presented in Fig. 9-10. These results indicate that light and medium work result in a decrease in caloric intake and in body weight and that heavy and very heavy work result in an increase in caloric intake, but body weight remained constant.

It was emphasized previously that the start of obesity for many persons has been associated with a decline in activity. A professional or college athlete in

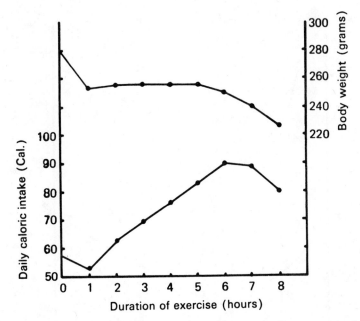

Fig. 9-9. Relationship between food intake, energy expenditure, and body weight. (Adapted from Mayer.[18])

training usually has very little trouble maintaining his weight, despite the fact that he usually eats all the food that he wants to. Yet many athletes do not maintain their activity level or do not decrease their food intake when they retire and so experience a problem controlling their weight. This is a problem also encountered by many individuals when they finish school and go to work. If their job is sedentary or inactive, they tend to exercise less but continue to eat as much as ever. The result, of course, is that they increase their weight very rapidly.

Johnson, Burke, and Mayer,[12] compared systematically both the caloric intake and activity level in carefully paired groups of obese and normal-weight school girls. The time spent by the obese girls participating in any type of exercise was less than half that spent by the nonobese girls. The remaining time spent by the obese group was used for "nonactive" activities. The caloric intake was higher in the nonobese group than in the obese group.

Cristakis[4] presents information showing how many minutes of certain selected activities are necessary to "balance out" the caloric value of certain common foods. A partial listing of his information is presented in Table 9-12. The numbers in the activity columns refer to the number of minutes that the activity must be performed to "balance out" the caloric content of each serving of food. For example, one large apple contains 101 Calories. This table indicates that to use an equivalent number of Calories one would either have to read for 56 minutes, bowl for 23 minutes, play golf for 20 minutes, walk for

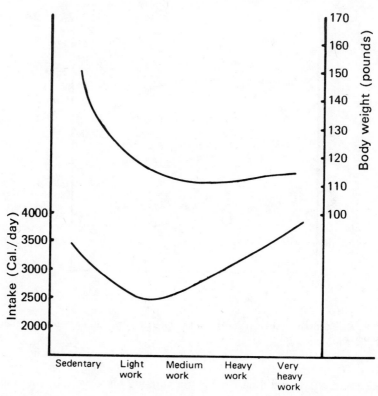

Fig. 9-10. Body weight and caloric intake as related to physical activity in man. (Adapted from Mayer.[18])

Table 9-12. Balance between caloric intake of selected foods and caloric expenditure of selected activities

Type of food	Calories per serving	Read-ing	Bowl-ing	Golf	Walk-ing	Tennis	Sleep-ing
Large apple	101	56	23	20	20	14	87
Boiled egg	77	43	17	15	15	11	66
Bread and butter	78	43	18	16	16	11	67
Two strips bacon	96	53	22	19	19	14	82
One glass beer	114	63	26	23	23	16	98
One glass milk	166	92	38	33	32	23	142
Cheese pizza	180	100	41	36	35	25	154
T-bone steak	235	131	53	47	45	33	201
Hamburger	350	194	80	70	67	49	300
Strawberry shortcake	400	222	91	80	77	56	343

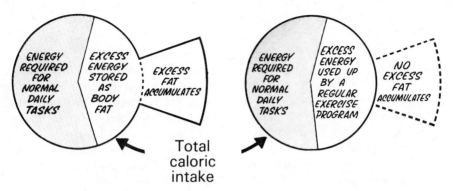

Fig. 9-11. Relationship between exercise, food intake, and accumulation of body fat. Either of the above two situations may apply to each individual. In each case the large circle represents the total caloric intake. It can be seen that if the excess energy is not used by participation in regular exercise, excess fat will accumulate. (Drawing by Eugene Sinervo; adapted from Royal Canadian Air Force Physical Fitness Program.)

20 minutes, play tennis for 14 minutes, or sleep for 87 minutes. The figures contained in this table are applicable to a person weighing 150 pounds.

The part that exercise can play in weight control is summarized in Fig. 9-11, which demonstrates very clearly the fact that activity burns up extra calories that would otherwise be stored as excess fat in the body. The more vigorous the activity, the more Calories are used up. It is important to realize, however, that activity does not have to be continuous to result in a loss in weight. The total amount of work will determine the number of Calories used.

Diet as a means to weight control

Most of the American adult population rely solely on various diets as a means to weight control. Each week we read of new diets that guarantee one to lose a certain amount of weight or a given number of inches from various areas of the body. Research has shown that over 9.5 million Americans are on diets at any given time during the year, whereas an additional 16.4 million indicate that they are watching their weight. A further 26.1 million indicate that they are "concerned" about their waistlines.[23]

In the same article the following summary of the effects of diet on weight control is presented:

> The 79 million American adults who are overweight today have more than their excess pounds in common. One central fact of their lives is that many millions of them will soon be going on yet another remarkable new diet. Chances are that this regimen will offer to relieve the duties of the burden of counting Calories. It will not cause hunger pangs. It will enable its adherents to lose precisely as many unsightly pounds as they choose. Unhappily, this promising new diet will be just that: promising. It may turn out to be damaging to the dieter's health, and it is practically guaranteed not to have any lasting effect on his or her overweight problem.[23]

Evidence is available to show that diets are successful with only a small percentage of persons. One study showed that out of every 100 who were concerned enough about weight control to see their doctor, only 7% actually attained their desired weight and only 2% were able to maintain this for a period of one year. The reason why diets are not more successful is that they cause an imbalance in the food intake. For example, a low carbohydrate diet may contain as much as 70% of daily Calories from fats. Apart from being damaging to a person's health, eating the same kinds of food each day becomes monotonous, and as a result most people do not maintain a diet for more than one or two months at the most. Usually, once they go off the diet, they put the weight back on again quickly.

What is necessary for weight control is a permanent change in daily eating habits, so that a person reduces his caloric intake and increases his caloric expenditure until a negative energy balance is established.

In summary, the following can be said as to the effects of diets:

1. Diets are a successful means of controlling weight for only a small percentage of persons.
2. Certain diets may result in a reduction in weight but at the same time may be damaging to one's health.
3. Most diets create an imbalance in the food intake, and therefore few individuals adhere to them for any length of time.
4. There are few new diets.
5. A diet will be successful only if a negative energy balance exists within the body.

SUMMARY

Basically, exercise does not use a large number of Calories. A 10- to 15-minute exercise program may use only 140 to 200 Calories. Comparing this to the caloric value of a slice of bread—75 Calories—or a piece of pie—250 Calories—one can see that a very small amount of food is the equivalent of a considerable amount of exercise. Those who exercise regularly should not be lulled into believing that if they are exercising 30 minutes a day, they can eat as much as they wish.

An individual certainly can use additional Calories by increasing his daily physical activity level, by climbing three flights of stairs four times a day rather than riding the elevator, by walking instead of riding, and by taking time to exercise regularly. The important point is that a man with a daily expenditure of 3,000 Calories will slowly lose weight if he takes in less than 3,000 Calories a day and will gain weight if he eats more than 3,000 Calories per day. Because a pound of fat is the equivalent of about 4,000 Calories, changes in caloric intake or caloric expenditure do not usually result in *rapid* weight fluctuations. Significant changes in weight are a result of a more prolonged reduction in food, together with an increase in caloric expenditure. Mayer summarizes the situation as follows:

Inactivity is the most important factor explaining the frequency of "creeping" overweight in modern Western societies. The regulation of food intake was never designed to adapt to the highly mechanized sedentary conditions of modern life. Adaptation to these conditions without development of obesity means that either the individual will have to step up his activity or that he will be mildly or acutely hungry all his life. The first alternative is difficult, especially as present conditions in the United States offer little inducement to walking and are often poorly organized as regards facilities for adult exercise. But if the first alternative of stepping up activity is difficult, it is well to remember that the second alternative, lifetime hunger, is so much more difficult to rely on.[18]

Diet alone is a much slower method for reducing weight than if combined with a good exercise program. It should be realized that this method of relying only on a diet is successful with a small percentage of persons and that many of these diets create such an imbalance in food intake that they may be quite hazardous to the individual's health.

REFERENCES

1. Allsen, P. E., Harrison, J. M., and Vance, B.: Fitness for life: an individualized approach, Dubuque, Iowa, 1975, Wm. C. Brown Company, Publishers.
2. Bronstein, I. P., et al.: Obesity in childhood, American Journal of Diseases of Children **63**:238, 1942.
3. Brozek, J., and Keys, A.: Relative body weight, age and fatness, Geriatrics **8**:70, 1953.
4. Christakis, G.: An anti-coronary club for prudent men. In The healthy life, New York, 1966, Time, Inc., p. 76.
5. Consolazio, C. F., et al.: Physiologic measurements of metabolic functions in man, New York, 1963, McGraw-Hill Book Company.
6. Corbin, C. B., et al.: Concepts in physical education, Dubuque, Iowa, 1970, Wm. C. Brown Company, Publishers.
7. Cundiff, D. E.: Fundamentals of physical fitness, Dubuque, Iowa, 1974, Kendall/Hunt Publishing Company, p. 127.
8. Garn, S. M., and Harper, R. V.: Fat accumulation and weight gain in adult males, Human Biology **27**:39, 1955.
9. Green, J. A.: Clinical studies of the etiology of obesity, American Internal Medicine **12**:1797, 1939.
10. Hickman, C. P.: Health for college students, Englewood Cliffs, N.J., 1963, Prentice-Hall, Inc., p. 208.
11. Hockey, R., Ritter, R., and Watson, R.: Evaluation of current physical fitness standards for freshman students enrolled at Northern Michigan University. Unpublished paper, Marquette, 1968, University of Northern Michigan.
12. Johnson, M. L., Burke, B. S., and Mayer, J.: Caloric intake in relation to energy output, American Journal of Clinical Nutrition **4**:231, 1956.
13. Johnson, P. B.: So you really want to lose weight, Toledo, Ohio, 1972, University of Toledo Press.
14. Johnson, R. E.: Exercise and weight control, a statement prepared for the committee on Exercise and Physical Fitness of the American Medical Association and the President's Council of Physical Fitness, Urbana, Aug., 1967, University of Illinois.

15. Keys, A., and Brozek, J.: Body fat in adult men, Physiological Reviews **33:**245, 1953.
16. Mayer, J.: Exercise and weight control. In Exercise and fitness, Chicago, 1960, The Athletic Institute, p. 110.
17. Mayer, J.: Obesity diagnosis, Postgraduate Medicine **25:**469, 1959.
18. Mayer, J.: Overweight: causes, cost, and control, Englewood Cliffs, N.J., 1968, Prentice-Hall, Inc.
19. Melograno, V., and Klinzing, J. E.: An orientation to total fitness, Dubuque, Iowa, 1974, Kendall Hunt Publishing Company, p. 127.
20. Metropolitan Life Insurance Co.: Overweight, its significance and prevention, New York, 1963, p. 31.
21. Rony, H. R.: Obesity and leanness, Philadelphia, 1940, Lea & Febiger.
22. Willoughby, D. P.: An anthropometric method for arriving at the optimal proportions of the body in the adult individual, Research Quartery **3:**48, 1932.
23. Wyden, P., and Wyden, B.: Why diet and exercise fads won't turn your fatness into fitness. In The healthy life, New York, 1966, Time, Inc.

Name _____   Date _____

Day and hour laboratory section meets _____

Laboratory instructor _____

DAILY CALORIC EXPENDITURE

Date _____   Day 1 (weekday)   Body weight _____

Activity	Minutes of participation	Cal/min/lb	Calories expended*

Date _____   Day 2 (weekend)   Body weight _____

Activity	Minutes of participation	Cal/min/lb	Calories expended*

Total Calories used per day _____   Total Calories used per day _____

*To calculate this, multiply cal/min/lb by the number of minutes of participation and then by your body weight.

Name _____   Date _____

Day and hour laboratory section meets _____

Laboratory instructor _____

DAILY CALORIC INTAKE

Day 1 (weekday)   Body weight _____

Date _____

Time of day	Type of food	Amount	Calories

Total Calories consumed per day _____

Day 2 (weekend)   Body weight _____

Date _____

Time of day	Type of food	Amount	Calories

Total Calories consumed per day _____

Fill in totals on following page.

Name _____ Date _____

Day and hour laboratory section meets _____

Laboratory instructor _____

SUMMARY SHEET FOR OVERWEIGHT AND BODY FAT EVALUATION

Height _____ inches Weight _____ pounds

Percent body fat _____ Percent overweight (height-weight charts) _____

Desirable weight (Willoughby Method) _____

Calculated energy balance (positive or negative) _____

Average caloric expenditure (average of day 1 and day 2) _____

Average caloric intake (average of day 1 and day 2) _____

Skinfold measurements

Men		**Women**	
Chest	_____	Iliac crest	_____
Abdomen	_____	Triceps	_____
Triceps	_____		

— —   **1.** Many diseases are attributable to lack of sufficient activity.

— —   **2.** The benefits of exercise are permanent.

— —   **3.** Without sufficient activity the body begins to deteriorate and possibly becomes more susceptible to certain illnesses and disease.

— —   **4.** Training decreases the oxygen requirement for work.

— —   **5.** Regular exercise has been shown to reduce the resting heart rate.

— —   **6.** If a trained and an untrained subject perform the same work task, the trained person will exhibit a higher heart rate.

— —   **7.** People who have desk jobs are more susceptible to low back pain than active workers.

— —   **8.** Low back pain is often the result of muscular deficiency.

— —   **9.** Physically active people are able to recover from a heart attack more frequently than sedentary people because collateral circulation is developed more.

— —   **10.** Exercise may reduce the free fatty acids and other lipids circulating in the blood.

chapter 10
Exercise and health

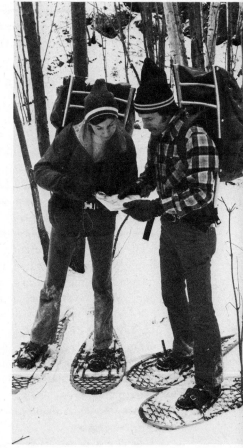

The necessity for regular exercise and its relationship to health is emphasized by Dr. Joseph Wolffe of the Valley Forge Heart Research Institute.

> It is imperative that the total population become aware of the urgent need and importance of physical exercise and health education as an important factor in the prevention of disease and attainment of TOTAL fitness. Not as an added feature, but as an integral part of living and education for living. Education for fitness from earliest childhood is a vital step in preventive medicine. The physician, the educator, the molder of the mind have the obligation to work as a team, to fuse their knowledge and their wisdom into a mobilization of popular opinion and conviction that the prolongation of a useful life depends upon how we use our bodies and brains.[17]

Kraus and Raab[10] suggest that this country is afflicted by a variety of pathological conditions that they classify as hypokinetic diseases—diseases attributable in a major or minor degree to lack of exercise. They further indicate that these diseases result in a reduction of earning power, early invalidism, and widespread mortality from functional and degenerative cardiovascular derangements.

PERSONAL BENEFITS OF REGULAR EXERCISE

Many students are interested in the reasons they should exercise regularly and in knowing what benefits can be derived from regular participation in a well-designed exercise program. Such a program should enable each student to achieve and maintain an adequate level of physical fitness, with which the following advantages are associated.

1. Feeling better physically and mentally. The student will have additional energy available so that the tasks and responsibilities of daily living will not drain him of his energy supply.

2. The ability to perform more work and recover faster following strenuous work. The American population has been described as lazy. To many people, life simply consists of putting in a day's work, coming home completely exhausted, eating dinner, and lying in the easy chair watching television or reading the paper. Many of these people are too tired to become involved in any recreational or family activities. With an increase in the level of physical fitness, they are able not only to perform more work before becoming fatigued but also to recover much faster after these tasks and will therefore have an increased margin of safety if called on to meet unforeseen circumstances. The increase in energy available is brought about by an increase in the efficiency of the body with regard to the use of oxygen. The body is able to use more oxygen and make more oxygen available to the working muscles. In this way the available energy is increased.

3. Improved personal appearance. There seems to be a direct relationship between personal appearance and one's physical fitness level. Most of us look better when we are physically fit than we do when we are unfit. Regular participation in a well-designed exercise program can play a very important part in weight control, which, of course, contributes toward the improvement of per-

sonal appearance. Not only does regular exercise help to reduce weight but it can reduce the percentage of body fat, increase the muscle tone, and through muscular development may result in improvement of posture.

4. Increased enjoyment of life. Various forms of exercise provide fun and enjoyment for many people. Different activities provide an opportunity for increasing a person's interest in life, allow one to meet new people, and to benefit from the out-of-doors. The person who takes time to develop his physical fitness level will enjoy life, for enjoyment of life depends more on a person's physical condition than on any other single factor. It is common knowledge that conditions such as headaches, fatigue, or illness are associated with a certain degree of discomfort. Some concern and attention for the development of good health and physical fitness will enhance the possibility of freedom from discomfort, which in turn makes living more enjoyable.

5. Decrease in the incidence of certain common health complaints and disorders. A gradual and progressive exercise program can produce a general resistance to certain common health complaints or illness. Cureton[4] has shown that when an active group of adult male subjects, ranging from 26 to 60 years of age was compared to a similar but inactive group, various differences were observed between the groups with regard to the incidence of certain health complaints. These results are summarized in Fig. 10-1. It can clearly be seen that the active group of men had a lower incidence of fatigue, body fat, headaches, hemorrhoids, and eye trouble.

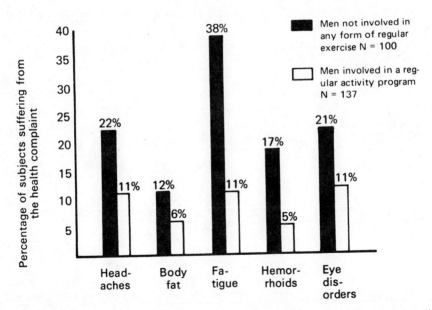

Fig. 10-1. Comparison between an active and an inactive group with regard to the incidence of certain health complaints. (Data from Cureton.[4])

6. Increased relaxation and mental alertness. Through regular exercise it has been shown that a student can relax more, concentrate for longer periods of time, and usually sleep better at night.

The preceding list should motivate students to exercise more. Most of us would like to feel better and look better and be able to enjoy life more by having more energy to participate in the activities we enjoy.

EFFECTS OF REGULAR EXERCISE ON HEART AND CIRCULATORY SYSTEM

Many other changes occur that are related to the heart and circulatory system. Some of these changes result in definite health benefits.

Increased heart efficiency

Karvonen[9] indicates that "the best pump is the pump that is most able to increase its performance and that functionally the best heart is the heart that can increase its output the most." It is usually the functional ability of the heart and circulatory system that is the limiting factor in heavy, prolonged work. The production of energy requires oxygen, and therefore the ability of the body to process and deliver sufficient oxygen to the working muscles is of primary importance. The trained heart is able to provide more oxygen because it is more efficient.

A trained heart is able to do the same amount of work with less effort. Through regular training the size of the heart may increase. This is often referred to as cardiac hypertrophy, or simply athlete's heart. This occurs because the heart, like any other muscle in our body, grows stronger and thicker if exercised properly. Many athletes involved in endurance events, such as long distance running, rowing, swimming, and wrestling, have hearts that are much larger than normal. These hearts reach a considerable weight and have a very large volume. The muscular walls are much thicker than those of the normal heart and are therefore stronger and more efficient. Each time such a heart contracts it does so with more force and thus has a larger stroke volume. With this larger stroke volume the trained heart is able to circulate the same amount of blood as the untrained heart, but it does not have to beat so frequently to achieve the same level.

Table 10-1. Comparison of stroke volume, cardiac output, and heart rate between a trained and untrained subject

	Stroke volume during exercise	*Cardiac output required to perform a standardized task*	*Heart rate necessary to achieve desired cardiac output*
Untrained	120 ml	21.5 liters/min	180
Trained	200 ml	21.5 liters/min	107

At rest the stroke volume of the untrained subject is approximately 70 ml. With a resting heart rate of 70 beats per minute there would be a cardiac output of 4,900 ml, which is the equivalent of 4.9 liters. For a highly trained subject the average stroke volume may be approximately 100 ml. To circulate the same amount of blood as the untrained subject, his heart need beat only 49 times per minute.

During exercise the differences between the trained and untrained subjects are much greater. The data from Williams[16] are summarized in Table 10-1.

Due to the large difference between the stroke volume of the trained (200 ml) and the untrained subjects (120 ml), the heart rate that is necessary to circulate the same amount of blood will be much higher in the untrained subject (180) than in the trained subject (107).

An increase in the size of the heart with training may therefore be associated with (1) an increase in stroke volume, (2) a decrease in resting heart rate, and (3) a decrease in the maximal heart rate attained during a standardized task.

A trained heart can produce more work before reaching the maximal heart rate. The maximal heart rate attained will be approximately the same for the trained and the untrained subject; however, the trained person will be able to perform more work before reaching the maximal heart rate (Fig. 10-2). It can clearly be seen that if 180 is the maximal heart rate, the subject could run

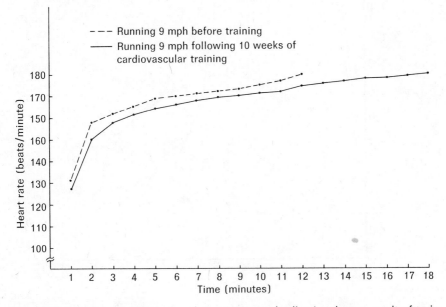

Fig. 10-2. Heart rate changes in relation to a standardized task as a result of training. With training the subject can run for 18 minutes at a speed of 9 mph before reaching 180 beats/minute, whereas before training it took only 12 minutes to reach the critical heart rate.

for only 12 minutes when not conditioned but could run for approximately 18 minutes as a result of training before reaching 180 beats per minute.

A trained heart can recover much faster following the performance of a task. The heart rate changes associated with regular participation in an exercise program have been demonstrated in a number of studies. Brouha[1] carefully examined the changes that occur in the exercise and recovery heart rates during the performance of a standardized task. These results are presented in Fig. 10-3. Despite the fact that the same work task was performed each time, the maximal heart rate attained during the training season was 10 beats lower than it was before the training began. Recovery after the task was much faster as a result of training. These changes resulting from increased heart efficiency were evident in a study by Skinner, Halloszy, and Cureton,[15] who studied the

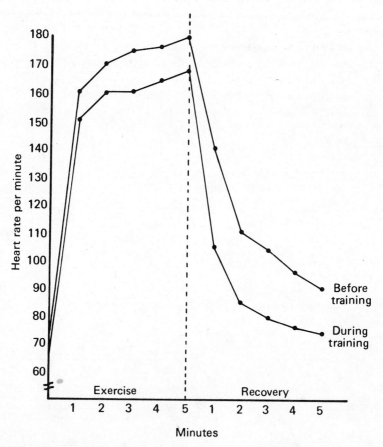

Fig. 10-3. Effect of training on the heart rate response to a standard amount of exercise. Note that there was a decrease from 180 to 170 in the maximal heart rate and that the heart rate returned to "normal" much quicker as a result of training. (Adapted from Brouha.[1])

effects of a 6-month program of endurance exercises on the cardiovascular system. Fifteen subjects were used, ranging from 35 to 55 years of age. The program consisted of progressive endurance training exercises as developed by Cureton.[4] Each subject participated a minimum of 3 days per week for approximately 45 minutes per day. Three of the endurance tests utilized were as follows:

1. A *mile run,* in which the subject attempts to run the distance in the shortest possible time
2. A *treadmill run,* in which the subject runs on the treadmill at 7 mph and 8.6% grade for as long as he can
3. A *5-minute step test,* in which the subject steps up to and down from a 17-inch bench at the rate of 30 steps per minute

The changes that occurred as a result of this program are presented in Table 10-2. These results indicate the following:

1. There was a marked decrease in the time taken to run a mile.
2. More work could be performed before reaching the maximal heart rate on the treadmill run despite the fact that the maximal heart rate was approximately the same each time.
3. After the performance on the 5-minute step test, which was a standardized task, there was a significant decrease in the heart rate as a result of training.

A reduced resting heart rate means more rest for the heart and less stress placed upon the heart. To find resting heart rates ranging from 40 to 55 beats per minute in trained subjects is not uncommon. When compared to the average resting heart rate for untrained subjects, which is approximately 70 beats per minute, this rate is very low. The heart of a trained subject at rest performs considerably less work than that of the average person. It is possible with regular training for a subject to reduce his resting heart rate from 70 to 50 beats per minute. Such a reduction would cause his heart to beat 28,800 times less each day. This would result in a significant reduction in the amount of work that the heart must perform. All these changes associated with training produce an increase in the efficiency of the heart. In simple terms, increased efficiency of the heart means (1) more work can be performed before becom-

Table 10-2. Effects of a 6-month program of endurance exercises on the mile run, the treadmill run performance, and the 5-minute step test

Test	*Initial result*	*Final result*	*Change*
Mile run (time)	531 sec	456 sec	− 75 sec
Treadmill run			
Time to exhaustion	118 sec	238 sec	+120 sec
Postexercise heart rate	178 beats/min	179 beats/min	+ 1 beat/min
5-minute step test			
Postexercise heart rate	176 beats/min	165 beats/min	− 11 beats/min

ing fatigued, (2) the same amount of work can be performed with less stress on the heart, (3) recovery will occur faster after the performance of a task, and (4) the heart will rest more.

Increased coronary blood supply and capillary development

The supply of blood to the heart muscle itself is most important. It was shown in Chapter 2 that there are tiny arteries, known as coronary arteries, that carry the blood supply to the heart muscle. Mellerowicz[12] indicates that these coronary arteries are extended roughly in proportion to the muscular development of the heart. This means that as a result of regular exercise these arteries will become larger.

Most forms of cardiovascular disease have their beginning with atherosclerosis, which is defined as a narrowing of the arteries caused by formation of fat deposits on the inner layer. A gradual enlargement of these arteries is beneficial, since it is more difficult for a blood clot to lodge in an enlarged artery. The date of Pétren, Sjöstrand, and Sylvén[14] indicate that the capillarization of the trained heart muscle is increased. Not only do the capillaries in the heart increase, but evidence shows that regular exercise will result also in an increase in the number of capillaries throughout the body. This allows for a more efficient exchange of gases and allows the body to *use* more of the oxygen that is available. This is one possible explanation as to why maximal oxygen intake increases with training. Of course, the more oxygen a person can use, the more energy he has available when stress is placed on the system.

Increased development of collateral circulation

If a blood clot lodges in a coronary artery, part of the heart muscle is deprived of its blood supply, unless there is an alternate pathway for the blood to travel. These alternate vessels, which may be available to direct the blood around the blocked artery, are referred to as *collateral vessels.* Collateral circulation simply means a new source of blood supply for a certain portion of the heart muscle. Newly formed blood vessels may spurt out from above and below the obstructed area, or tiny blood vessels that connect various branches of the arteries may be already developed. A classical study by Eckstein[6] showed that in trained dogs the collateral development was much greater than in untrained dogs when the coronary blood supply was restricted. Although this study used dogs, it would appear that a similar relationship exists with humans.[18]

Autopsies have revealed that a number of persons who have died of some disease not connected with the heart have had one or more segments of the coronary arteries completely occluded. Apparently collateral circulation can be developed to such an extent that it completely takes over if the major artery becomes blocked.[13]

It was shown in Chapter 3 that the incidence of death after a heart attack is much higher in an inactive group than in an active group of subjects. The more active a person, the greater his chance of surviving an initial heart attack. The increase in collateral circulation as a result of exercise presents a possible explanation. If these alternate pathways are adequately developed, the heart may continue functioning normally when one of the coronary arteries becomes blocked. If collateral circulation is developed with exercise, then it can be said that exercise is helpful in reducing the incidence of heart disease.

Increased fat tolerance

When one ingests a high fat meal, a certain amount of this fat passes through the bloodstream and is deposited in the liver or stored as adipose tissue. This process is referred to as lipid metabolism. The efficiency with which one clears these lipids from the bloodstream is termed fat tolerance. A person who clears fat quickly from the blood is said to have high fat tolerance, whereas poor fat tolerance refers to a delayed clearing of fat from the bloodstream. Exercise after a high fat meal has been shown to reduce the level of fat in the bloodstream and thus increase the fat tolerance. A study by Cantone[3] demonstrates the effect that exercise has on the lipid metabolism (Fig. 10-4). This study shows that not only is fat cleared much more quickly from the bloodstream as a result of exercise, but that the maximal amount of lipids in the blood is also reduced considerably. When one considers that it is fatty deposits that contribute to atherosclerosis, the health benefits associated with the quick clearing of fat from the bloodstream appear obvious.

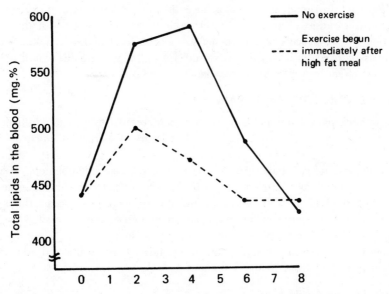

Fig. 10-4. Effect of exercise on lipid metabolism. Note that when the exercise was begun immediately after a high-fat meal, the lipids were cleared quickly. (Adapted from Cantone.[3])

Reduction of obesity and overweight

Regular participation in a well-designed activity program has been shown to result in the reduction of excess fat and weight. The effects of exercise on these two variables are discussed in detail in Chapter 9.

Excess weight and excess fat can affect the circulatory system in two ways. They can cause extra stress to be placed on the heart and can also result in an increase in blood pressure. By reducing excess weight and fat, a person is reducing two risk factors associated with an increased incidence of cardiovascular disease.

Reduced clotting ability of the blood

The part that a blood clot plays in heart disease already has been discussed. Within the blood is a substance called fibrin, which is a protein necessary for the formation of a blood clot. Two systems concerned with fibrin operate within the body: (1) coagulation, concerned with the formation of fibrin, and (2) fibrinolysis, concerned with the breakdown of fibrin. These systems operate in opposition to one another to maintain an equilibrium within the body.

In a well-controlled study, Burt, Blyth, and Rierson[2] studied the effects of exercise on both these systems. They found that exercise shortens the blood clotting time approximately 19%, which means that blood clots faster. However, exercise also speeds up the process of fibrinolysis by 69%. This means that blood clots are dissolved much faster. Since the increase was much greater for fibrinolysis than it was for coagulation, it was shown that exercise results in the overall reduction of the clotting ability of the blood.

There is also good reason to believe that since fibrin is a sticky protein substance, it causes other substances to adhere to the vessel walls, thus contributing to the process of atherosclerosis. If the level of fibrin in the bloodstream is reduced with exercise, it would appear as though this would have a beneficial effect by reducing the incidence of atherosclerosis.

EXERCISE AND LOW BACK PAIN

Low back pain is one of the most common complaints among adults in the United States today. It results in many lost hours of work and much discomfort.

Kraus and Raab[10] have classified low back pain as a hypokinetic disease, which they define as a disease caused by insufficient activity. This is in agreement with Feffer,[7] a well-known orthopedic surgeon, who states that "the increase in the incidence of low back pain is related to the increasingly sedentary life we lead. We simply do not get enough exercise."

Low back pain is a "disease" that occurs fairly early in life and appears to be most prevalent from 25 to 35 years of age.

Causes of low back pain

The major cause of low back pain is improper muscular development. The development and maintenance of muscle function is dependent upon its use.

The strength of a muscle is directly related to the amount of work that it does. As a muscle works against a resistance, the strength of that muscle will increase. If the muscle does not perform any work, a loss of strength will result. In an inactive person many of the large muscle groups are not used frequently enough. They therefore lack sufficient strength to maintain the correct body alignment, which is one of their specific tasks.

Poor abdominal development is one of the most common causes of low back pain. The pelvis should be tipped up in the front, but if the abdominal muscles are weak, they are unable to exert sufficient pressure to keep the pelvis in place, and it drops down in the front, causing a forward pelvic tilt. This in turn causes the vertebrae in the lower back region to be slightly displaced, and their articular processes press against one another, causing the ache in the lower area of the back.[1]

Another group of muscles associated with low back pain is commonly referred to as the *hamstring muscle group*. This group consists of three muscles —the *biceps femoris*, the *semimembranosus* and the *semitendinosus* muscles.

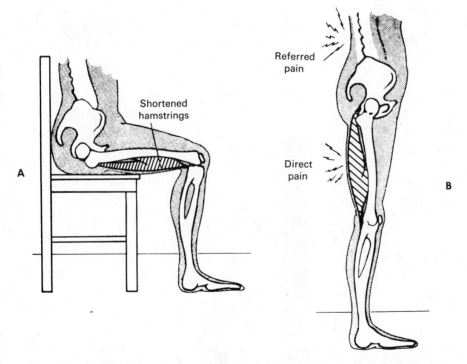

Fig. 10-5. A, Position of the hamstring muscle group in relation to the bone structure when in a sitting posture. If much of the time is spent sitting, this muscle group may become much shorter than it should be. **B,** Effect that a shortening of the hamstring muscles has on the pelvis, when one assumes an upright standing position. (Drawings by Eugene Sinervo; adapted from Johnson et al.[8])

All three of these muscles lie along the posterior aspect of the thigh and all are associated with movement at both the hip and the knee joints.

The difficulty experienced by most persons in touching the toes with the fingertips without bending the knees is caused by the fact that the hamstring muscles are often not long enough to permit such extreme stretching.[10] This shortening of the hamstring muscle group will often occur in those who spend a large amount of time in a sitting position (Fig. 10-5, *A*). If these muscles are not given any stretching exercises, and if they are constantly held in positions that tend to shorten them, they become adjusted to this position. When a person assumes the standing position, both the knee and hip joints are fully extended (Fig. 10-5, *B*). If the hamstring muscles are shorter than they should be, this will cause both direct pain in the immediate area of the muscles and referred pain in the lower back region. Kraus and Raab state that:

> In our civilized cities we lead the lives of caged animals. We have no opportunity to move, no chance to respond to outside irritations. Besides, most of us are burdened by emotional problems, adding to the need for release. Since our civilization does not permit the natural responses of fight or flight, and since we do not have vicarious outlets by heavy exercise, tension is stored up in our muscles. This constant tension shortens the muscles and deprives them of elasticity. Once this muscle tightness has reached a sufficiently high level, and lack of physical activity has weakened our tense muscles, the stage is set for the first episode of back pain.[10]

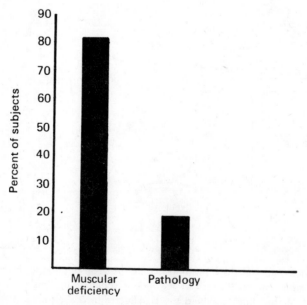

Fig. 10-6. Causes of low back pain. Note that over 80% of low back pain is due to muscular deficiency. (Adapted from Kraus and Raab.[10])

Kraus and Raab present evidence indicating that over 80% of low back pain is caused by muscular deficiency. Their results are summarized in Fig. 10-6. The test that was used to evaluate these patients was the Kraus-Weber test, which is a test of *minimal* muscular strength and flexibility.[11]

Kraus-Weber test

The Kraus-Weber test is a simple six-item test that can be used effectively to identify individuals who are likely to suffer from low back pain in the future. It should be stressed that this test measures only minimal muscular strength and flexibility. Following is a description of each of the six items that make up this test.

1. *Straight-leg sit-up.* The subject assumes a supine position (faceup) on the floor with hands held behind the neck. With legs straight and feet held down, he simply rolls up into a sitting position, keeping his hands behind his neck. This is a test for minimal strength of the abdominal muscles and also the psoas major muscle.

2. *Bent-leg sit-up.* The subject assumes a supine position on the floor with hands held behind the neck, knees bent, and bottoms of the feet flat on the floor. With feet held down and hands remaining behind the neck, he again rolls up into a sitting position. This is a test for minimal strength of the abdominal muscles.

3. *Forward leg lift.* The subject assumes a supine position on the floor with hands held behind the neck and legs extended. With legs straight, the feet are lifted 10 inches off the floor, and this position is held for 10 seconds. This test is designed to measure minimal strength of the lower abdominal muscles.

4. *Trunk lift.* The subject assumes a prone position (facedown) on the floor, with a pillow under his abdomen. With hands behind the neck and feet and hips held down, the subject raises his trunk and holds this position for 10 seconds. This is a test of minimal strength of the upper back muscles.

5. *Backward leg raise.* The subject again assumes a prone position over a pillow. With back and hips held, he must lift his legs and hold them off the ground for 10 seconds. This is a test of minimal strength of the lower back muscles.

6. *Toe touch.* The subject stands erect with legs straight and feet held together. He then reaches down slowly without forcing unnecessarily and touches the floor with his fingertips. This position is maintained for a period of 3 seconds. No jerking movements are allowed, and the legs must remain perfectly straight throughout. This is a test of the length of the hamstring muscle group.

Each student is evaluated on each of these items simply on a pass-fail basis. If a person cannot pass all six, he has failed the test. This classifies him as a potential sufferer of low back pain. This is the test that was given to a group of American and European children in 1952. Over 57% of the American children failed to pass one or more of the six items that make up this test. This could partly explain the high incidence of low back pain in this country today.

SUMMARY

Several of the changes that take place as a result of exercise could explain why there is a reduction in the incidence of cardiovascular disease associated with regular participation in a well-designed exercise program:

1. Increase in the efficiency of the heart
2. Increase in the coronary blood supply
3. Development of collateral circulation
4. Reduced resting heart rate, meaning more rest for the heart
5. Quicker clearance of fat from the bloodstream
6. Reduction in the clotting ability of the blood
7. Reduction in excess weight and fat
8. Reduction in systolic blood pressure

Associated with each of these changes is a possible explanation as to why regular exercise might reduce one's chances of suffering from some form of cardiovascular disease. An understanding of the material presented in this chapter should make it possible for a student to become aware of the relationship between each of these changes and cardiovascular disease.

Other changes that relate to the cardiovascular system resulting from regular exercise include the following:

1. An increase in the amount of hemoglobin and total blood volume, which would make it possible for the body to deliver more oxygen to the body
2. An increase in the efficiency of the lungs, which would allow them to process more air with less effort
3. An increase in the maximal amount of oxygen that the body is able to utilize

All the changes outlined in this chapter make it possible for a person to live a fuller and more productive life. An individual is able to perform more work before becoming fatigued or to perform the same amount of work with less physiological stress. Williams[16] summarizes the effects of training as follows: "The objective of training is to permit the performance of an activity with less disturbance to the internal environment and also to increase the activity potential of the individual."

In the discussion on physical fitness, it was indicated that a certain "minimal" level of muscular strength is necessary. Those persons who are unable to manage their own weight and to maintain adequate posture do not possess this "minimal" level of strength. Not meeting this level should indicate that the amount of physical activity of that individual is not sufficient to meet his demands.

Those persons who are potential candidates for low back pain are easy to determine. These individuals should include in their activity programs exercises that will reduce the likelihood of suffering from low back pain. Much time and money could be saved if one would take time to exercise regularly to alleviate low back pain, rather than trying to find alternate, easy short-cut methods, which really are nonexistent. A complete exercise program for alleviation of low back pain is presented in detail in Chapter 14.

REFERENCES

1. Brouha, L.: The effect of work on the heart. In Rosenbaum, F. F., and Belknap, E., editors: Work and the heart, New York, 1959, Paul B. Hoeber, Inc., p. 184.
2. Burt, J. J., Blyth, C. S., and Rierson, H. A.: Effects of exercise on the coagulation-fibrinolysis equilibrium, Journal of Sports Medicine and Physical Fitness 4:213, 1964.
3. Cantone, A.: Physical effort and its effect in reducing alimentary hyperlipaeminia, Journal of Sports Medicine and Physical Fitness 4:32, 1964.
4. Cureton, T. K.: Run for your life. In The healthy life, New York, 1966, Time, Inc., p. 35.
5. DiGennaro, J.: Individualized exercise and optimal physical fitness, Lea & Febiger, Philadelphia, 1974, p. 97.
6. Eckstein, R. W.: Effect of exercise and coronary artery narrowing on coronary collateral circulation, Circulation Research 5:230, 1957.
7. Feffer, H.: All about backache, Readers Digest, Dec. 1971, p. 203.
8. Johnson, P. B., et al.: Physical education—a problem solving approach to health and fitness, New York, 1966, Holt Rinehart and Winston, Inc.
9. Karvonen, M. J.: Effects of vigorous exercise on the heart. In Rosenbaum, F. F., and Belknap, E., editors: Work and the heart, New York, 1959, Paul B. Hoeber, Inc., p. 199.
10. Krause, H., and Raab, W.: Hypokinetic disease, Springfield, Ill., 1961, Charles C Thomas, Publisher, p. 8.
11. Krause, H., and Eisenmenger-Weber, S.: Quantitative tabulation of posture evaluation, based on structural and functional measurements, The Physiotherapy Review 26:235, 1946.
12. Mellerowicz, H.: The effect of training on heart and circulation and its importance in preventive cardiology. In Raab, W., editor: Prevention of ischemic heart disease, Springfield, Ill., 1966, Charles C Thomas, Publisher, p. 309.
13. Mozes, E. B.: Living beyond your heart attack, Englewood Cliffs, N.J., 1959, Prentice-Hall, Inc., p. 17.
14. Pétren, T., Sjöstrand, T., and Sylvén, B.: The influence of training on the capillarization of the heart and skeletal musculature, Arbeitsphysiologie 9:376, 1936.
15. Skinner, J. S., Halloszy, J. O., and Cureton, T. K.: Effects of a program of endurance exercises on physical work, American Journal of Cardiology 14:747, 1964.
16. Williams, J. G.: Medical aspects of sport and physical fitness, Oxford, 1965, Pergamon Press, p. 12.
17. Wolffe, J. B.: Prevention of disease through exercise and health education. In Health and fitness in the modern world, Chicago, 1961, The Athletic Institute, p. 75.
18. Zoll, P. M., et al.: Interarterial anastamoses in the human heart with particular reference to anemia and relative cardiac anoxia, Circulation 14:797, 1956.

chapter 11
Skill and motor ability

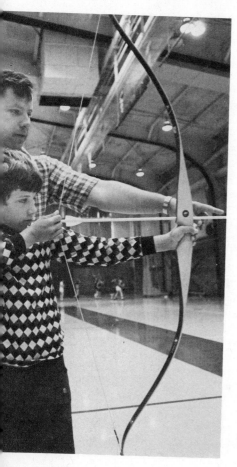

— —   **1.** Motor ability and physical fitness are synonymous terms.

— —   **2.** Football is an activity that should be stressed because it is a good carry-over activity.

— —   **3.** An increased skill level in an activity like handball will be likely to result in an increased heart rate during participation.

— —   **4.** No activities regardless of skill level will be as beneficial as running for the development of cardiovascular endurance.

— —   **5.** Agility is most important in swimming.

— —   **6.** The best measure of power is the 50-yard dash.

— —   **7.** Speed and reaction time are really the same.

— —   **8.** Athletes are superior to untrained subjects in reaction time.

— —   **9.** Reaction time is very important in wrestling.

— —   **10.** Balance may be defined as the ability to maintain the equilibrium of the body.

Participation in activities such as basketball, tennis, handball, and swimming can play an important part in the development of physical fitness. For this reason, developing one's skill level in several of these activities is important because the higher the person's skill level is in an activity, the more likely he is to be motivated to participate in it. We all enjoy doing the things we do well.

One of the major objectives of any physical education program is the development of a person's skill level. A person who performs a skill well is said to exhibit good motor ability. Motor ability can thus be defined as the skillful performance of a physical skill.

Each individual should make an attempt to become skillful in at least one activity and preferably in more than one. The types of activities that a person can enjoy and participate in later in life should be stressed in both high school and college physical education programs. These activities are often referred to as "lifetime" sports and include such activities as bowling, golf, archery, tennis, swimming, hunting, fishing, handball, and paddle ball.

In the selection of activities, some thought should be given to whether they can be used later in life and whether they will contribute to the development of physical fitness. Persons usually do not participate in such activities as basketball, baseball, and football later in life, and activities such as archery, volleyball, golf, hunting, and fishing have only minimal, if any, contributions to make toward the development of physical fitness. This is not to say that these are not good recreational activities. However, if a person can select an activity that he enjoys participating in and that will contribute toward the development of physical fitness, it is much better for him to participate in this

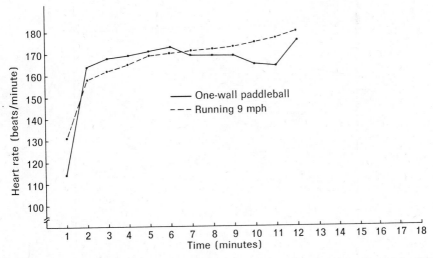

Fig. 11-1. Comparison of heart rate responses for running at 9 mph and participating in one-wall racquetball singles competition.

activity than in one that can be used only for recreational purposes. The heart rate response to running for 12 minutes at a rate of 9 miles per hour is presented in Fig. 11-1. Also presented is the obtained heart rate for the same subject during participation in badminton singles competition. It can clearly be seen that both of these activities elevate the heart rate considerably and can be used for the development of physical fitness.

It is also interesting to note that the higher the person's skill level as well as that of his opponent is in a particular sport, the greater energy expenditure is involved. In many instances this will result in a greater contribution of these activities to the development of cardiovascular endurance.

COMPONENTS OF MOTOR ABILITY

The six generally recognized components of motor ability are (1) agility, (2) power, (3) coordination, (4) speed, (5) reaction time, and (6) balance.

Agility

Agility may be defined as the ability to change direction accurately and quickly while moving rapidly. In some activities the ability to stop and start and to change direction quickly is much more important than in others. In sports such as basketball, badminton, handball, and tennis, agility is a most important factor. This may be measured by such tasks as the shuttle run and activities that require a quick change of direction.

Probably the most commonly used test for measuring this component is the

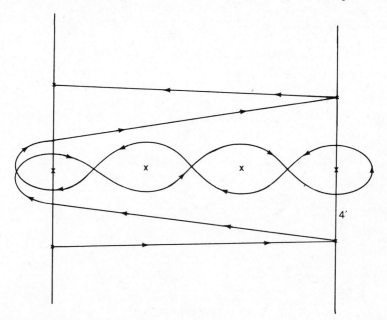

Fig. 11-2. Pattern to be followed for the agility run. Each of the four chairs or cones in the center line are placed 10 feet apart.

Illinois Agility Run.[1] The subject assumes a prone position with the hands beside the chest and forehead on the starting line. He jumps up at the starting signal and follows the zigzag pattern shown in Fig. 11-2.

The aim is to complete the pattern in the shortest possible time. Measurement is in terms of seconds and is recorded to the nearest tenth of a second from the starting signal until the subject crosses the finish line. The test must be taken with rubber soled gym shoes. Two trials are allowed, with at least 2 minutes of rest allowed between them.

The results for the test should be recorded:

Trial 1 _____ seconds

Trial 2 _____ seconds

Best trial _____ seconds

Power

Power is defined as the ability to exert a maximal contraction in one explosive act. It is sometimes referred to as explosive strength. It is dependent on two other factors—strength and speed. A good example of this is the shot put. In this event the participant combines strength and speed as they are coordinated into an explosive movement, with the maximal force being exerted as quickly as possible. The broad jump is another example of an activity in which power is most important. To a lesser degree it is important in the jump shot in basketball. This factor may be measured by the standing broad jump, the medicine ball put, or the jump-and-reach test. No matter what test is used for measuring this factor, the person is required to jump or project himself or some object either as far or as high as possible.[3]

For evaluating power, both the standing broad jump and the jump-and-reach test are good. Because of its ease of administration, the standing broad jump may be preferred over the jump-and-reach test. The standing broad jump measures explosive leg power, which is dependent on speed and strength. A starting line is marked on the floor, and the subject stands with feet apart and toes behind the starting line. He then flexes at the hips, knees, and ankles and, by swinging the arms, jumps as far forward as possible. Measurement is to the nearest inch, from the take-off line to the heel of the foot nearest the take-off line or any portion of the body nearer the line. Two trials are allowed.

The results for the standing broad jump should be recorded:

Trial 1 _____ inches

Trial 2 _____ inches

Best trial _____ inches

Coordination

Coordination can be defined as the integration of separate abilities into the smooth execution of a task. This may involve various parts of the body, such as eye-foot coordination, as in kicking a football, or hand-eye coordination, as in catching a tennis ball. An example might help to demonstrate exactly what is meant by coordination. Consider the breaststroke in swimming. A student can learn the arm stroke and the kick separately and usually very quickly. The most difficult aspect of this skill is learning how to combine these two parts so that maximum performance will result.

When two forces are added sequentially such as in this skill, the exact time that the second force is initiated is most important. If it is started too soon or too late, a decrease in performance will result. Adding this second force at the right time is an example of good coordination.

Coordination has often been referred to as a general motor ability. The reason is that no matter what activity is analyzed, various movements must be integrated if skilled performance is to be demonstrated. An increase in coordination will result in increased efficiency in the performance of the skill. Coordination is important in all activities.

In activities such as badminton and tennis, hand-eye coordination is very important. A good test to evaluate this component is the alternate-hand wall toss. Three tennis balls, a stop watch, and a smooth-surfaced wall are required for the administration of this test. The subject stands facing the wall, behind a 6-foot restraining line, with a ball held in the right hand. The two extra tennis balls are located in a container at the side of the right foot. At the starting signal the ball is tossed against the wall with an underhand motion and caught in the left hand. It is then thrown with the left hand and caught with the right hand. This movement is repeated as often as possible during a 30-second period. The number of successful catches completed in 30 seconds is counted. The ball must be thrown underhand and cannot be trapped against the body. The restraining line cannot be crossed. One minute of practice is allowed for each subject, followed by two trials.

The results for the alternate-hand wall toss should be recorded:

Trial 1 _____ repetitions

Trial 2 _____ repetitions

Best trial _____ repetitions

Speed and reaction time

Speed is defined as the quickness with which one is able to move his body from one point to another. The distance covered may vary, but in each instance the aim is to move from one point to another in the shortest possible time. Actually, the time taken to perform a task such as this also includes reaction time—defined as the time required to initiate a response to a specific stimulus.[4]

That speed of movement and the ability to react quickly are of great importance in many different activities is generally recognized. Athletic games and contests abound with illustrations of split-second responses to a stimulus. Keller[5] has shown that when 359 athletes were compared to 277 nonathletes, the athletes were superior to the nonathletes in speed and reaction time.

Another study by Tuttle and Westerlund[6] showed also that "outstanding" athletes were superior to "average" athletes in both speed and reaction time.

The sports in which speed and reaction time appear to be most important are baseball, basketball, football, and track. Participants in these sports have been shown to be quicker than participants in gymnastics, wrestling, and swimming.[5] Because of this, students who do not possess above average speed may have a greater chance of success in the latter three sports than in those of the other group.

Speed can be measured by how fast an individual can move from one point to another. Actually, any distance ranging from 10 to 100 yards can be used for determination of speed. The two distances most frequently used are 50 and 100 yards. Two trials should be given for whichever one of these two tests are used, and the results should be recorded:

_____ yard dash

Trial 1 _____ seconds

Trial 2 _____ seconds

Best trial _____ seconds

Reaction time is defined as the amount of time elapsing between a stimulus and the first movement initiated in response to it. To measure this component, generally one must use special equipment designed for the purpose. However, if a short distance is used for measuring speed, the time will reflect not only the subject's speed but also his reaction time, since both are included in the time taken to complete the performance.

Balance

Balance may be defined as ability to maintain the equilibrium of the body. The two types of balance are static and dynamic. With static balance the equilibrium is maintained in a fixed position, usually while standing on one foot. With dynamic balance the equilibrium must be maintained while performing some task. This might involve walking on a balance beam. The three basic factors that can influence balance are as follows:

1. The height of the center of gravity—the lower the center of gravity, the greater the balance and stability.
2. The size of the base of support—the larger the base of support, the greater the balance and stability.
3. The more nearly centered the line of gravity is to the center of the base of support, the greater the stability.

Balance is important in many different activities and is certainly a contributing factor to skillful performance.

Static balance. This involves any situation in which the body must produce stability and in which no movement takes place. A simple static balance test requires one to assume a diver's stance with the arms outstretched in front, standing on the toes, and with the eyes closed. The aim is to maintain this position as long as possible. This is also one of the items on the 18-item Illinois motor fitness test. To pass this item one must maintain the position for 20 seconds.[2]

Dynamic balance. This involves the maintenance of equilibrium while movement is involved. Available are many tests using the balance beam for evaluation of dynamic balance.

FACTORS THAT INFLUENCE SELECTION OF ACTIVITIES

Many factors influence a person when he decides which activities he will participate in. Van Huss et al.[7] list the following:

1. Present emotional needs
2. Present physical needs
3. Present social needs
4. Present interests
5. Future type of work
6. Future place of residence
7. Carry-over values
8. Present level of skills
9. Body type

These factors should be considered by each person, since they can help him to make a much wiser decision with regard to which activities will be most beneficial now and in the future.

REFERENCES

1. Adams, W. C., Haskell, W. L., Leigh, R. D., Hottinger, W. L., and Penny, W. J.: Foundations of physical activity, Champaign, Ill., Stipes Publishing Co., p. 131.
2. Cureton, T. K.: Run for your life. In The healthy life, New York, 1966, Time, Inc., p. 38.
3. Fleishman, E. A.: The structure and measurement of physical fitness, Englewood Cliffs, N.J., 1964, Prentice-Hall, Inc., p. 29.
4. Johnson, P. B., Updyke, W. F., Stolberg, D. C., and Schaefer, M.: Physical education—a problem solving approach to health and fitness, New York, 1966, Holt, Rinehart and Winston, Inc., p. 26.
5. Keller, L. F.: The relation of quickness of bodily movement to success in athletics, Research Quarterly **13:**146, 1942.
6. Tuttle, W. W., and Westerlund, J. A.: Relationship between running events in track and reaction time, Research Quarterly **2:**95, 1931.
7. Van Huss W., Niemeyer, R., Olson, H., and Friedrich, J.: Physical activity in modern living, ed. 2, Englewood Cliffs, N.J., 1969, Prentice-Hall, Inc., p. 173.

MOTOR ABILITY PROFILE CHART
Directions

Circle the score closest to the one obtained by you on each test. Connect the circles with a line so that comparisons may be made among the tests.

Men

Percentile rank	AGILITY Agility run (sec)	POWER Standing broad jump (inches)	COORDINATION Alternate-hand wall toss	SPEED 100-yard dash	SPEED 50-yard dash
95	15.0	104	38	11.8	6.1
90	15.6	101	36	12.2	6.2
80	16.3	96	33	12.6	6.4
70	16.8	92	31	12.9	6.5
60	17.2	90	30	13.1	6.6
50	17.6	87	28	13.4	6.8
40	18.0	84	26	13.7	6.9
30	18.4	82	25	13.9	7.0
20	18.9	78	23	14.2	7.1
10	19.6	73	20	14.6	7.5
5	20.2	70	18	15.0	7.7
Mean	17.6	87.0	28.0	13.4	6.8
SD	1.6	10.6	6.3	1.2	.8

Women

Percentile rank	AGILITY Agility run (sec)	POWER Standing broad jump (inches)	COORDINATION Alternate-hand wall toss	SPEED 50-yard dash
95	18.4	77	30	7.3
90	19.1	73	27	7.6
80	19.8	69	24	7.8
70	20.3	66	22	8.0
60	20.8	63	21	8.2
50	21.2	61	19	8.4
40	21.6	59	17	8.7
30	22.1	56	16	9.0
20	22.5	53	14	9.2
10	23.3	49	11	9.7
5	24.0	45	8	10.1
Mean	21.2	61.0	19.0	8.4
SD	1.7	9.5	6.5	.8

Name _____ Date _____

Day and hour laboratory section meets _____

Laboratory instructor _____

SUMMARY SHEET FOR MOTOR ABILITY TEST

Agility run
Trial 1 _____ seconds
Trial 2 _____ seconds
Best trial _____ seconds

Standing broad jump
Trial 1 _____ inches
Trial 2 _____ inches
Best trial _____ inches

Alternate-hand wall toss
Trial 1 _____ repetitions
Trial 2 _____ repetitions
Best trial _____ repetitions

_____ -yard dash
Trial 1 _____ seconds
Trial 2 _____ seconds
Best trial _____ seconds

T   F

___ ___ **1.** Any existing exercise program is good and can be used for the optimal development of physical fitness.

___ ___ **2.** One of the advantages of the aerobics program is that it is one of the few scientifically developed programs.

___ ___ **3.** In the aerobics program most activities are converted to a point system based on the amount of energy expenditure.

___ ___ **4.** Tennis is a good activity for the development of cardiovascular endurance.

___ ___ **5.** The aim of circuit training is simply to perform a series of calisthenics with rest periods in between.

___ ___ **6.** In circuit training each student is competing against each other student.

___ ___ **7.** Circuit training does not concentrate on the development of cardiovascular endurance.

___ ___ **8.** Progressive overload is built into the circuit training program.

___ ___ **9.** Jogging and running are synonymous terms.

___ ___ **10.** Low back pain exercises should aim at the development of the abdominal muscles and stretching of the hamstring muscle group.

___ ___ **11.** In the aerobics program the only way a person can earn the required number of points per week is through running, swimming, or riding a bike.

chapter 12
Existing exercise programs

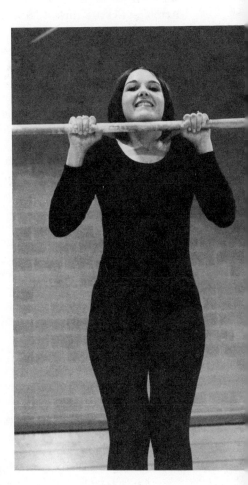

There are many different exercise programs that have been developed and that can be be used to develop and maintain an adequate level of physical fitness. Several of these programs will be summarized in this chapter. Students may wish to use these programs in their entirety or adjust the programs to meet their individual needs.

THE AEROBICS PROGRAM[2]

Many times it is of interest to know the individual's capacity for muscular work. This ability to sustain heavy, prolonged muscular work is dependent on the supply of necessary oxygen to the working muscles. *Aerobic work* is thus defined as work performed when sufficient oxygen can be supplied by the body to produce the necessary energy for the performance of the task. Aerobic tasks are those that usually can be maintained for at least 10 minutes and during the performance of which no true oxygen debt is incurred.

The program referred to as *Aerobics* was developed by Dr. Kenneth H. Cooper following four years of research using over 15,000 United States Air Force personnel. There really is nothing new concerning the activities that are included in this program, since it utilizes common everyday activities such as walking, running, tennis, and golf. What *is* new about the program is the point system that has been developed as a result of the research. This system allows an individual to equate different activities in terms of energy expenditure and, in this way, to determine *which kinds of activities are best* and also *how long he must participate* in an activity to attain the beneficial results.

This program appears to be designed specifically for the development of the cardiovascular system. A basic assumption underlying this program appears to be that if you develop the cardiovascular system, this will automatically result in the development of "adequate" levels of the other three components of physical fitness—strength, muscular endurance, and flexibility.

In the aerobics program, Cooper was able to equate performance on most activities and then convert this to a point system according to the amount of energy expenditure. The activities that are more strenuous than others were given a higher point value.

Procedures for initiating an aerobics program

Listed are certain procedures that must be followed in order that maximal benefits may be gained from this program:

1. Each participant must know exactly how long he needs to participate in any activity to gain a particular number of points. This is determined by consulting the charts presented by Cooper.
2. Each subject should earn 30 points per week by selecting the work level from any of the available activities. Subjects who have an initially low level of physical fitness should start out by earning only 10 or 15 points per week and increase this work load gradually.
3. A minimum of three or four workouts per week is necessary. To earn all 30 points in one exercise session is not acceptable.

4. An accurate record should be kept of the points earned each day.

5. Periodical evaluation of progress should be made. The 12-minute run test is presented for this purpose, and by periodic use of this a subject can easily measure his progress. This test, of course, can be used to earn points for any day that the subject chooses to use it.

Typical point values for activities

Cooper's findings indicate that the most beneficial activities are running, swimming, cycling, stationary running, handball, and basketball. The amount or rate of work that would need to be performed for several of these activities to achieve certain points is presented in Table 12-1.

His findings also indicated that activities such as weight lifting, calisthenics, and isometrics did not contribute to the development of cardiovascular endur-

Table 12-1. Point values for certain selected activities in the aerobics program

Running (time for 1 mile)	Running (time for 2 miles)	Handball or basketball*	Swimming (time for 400 yards)	Cycling (time for 3 miles)	Points
More than 20 min	—	Less than 8 min	—	18 min or longer	0
14½-20 min	40 min or longer	8 min	13½ min or longer	12-17 min	1
12-14½ min	29-40 min	15 min	10-13½ min	—	2
10-12 min	—	20 min	7-9 min	9-11 min	3
8-10 min	24-28 min	28 min	—	—	4
6½-8 min	—	35 min	Less than 7 min	Less than 9 min	5
Less than 6½ min	20-24 min	40 min	—	—	6

*The times for handball and basketball are for continuous activity and do not include breaks, etc.; must also be full court basketball.

Table 12-2. Point values for certain additional exercises in the aerobics program

Activity	Amount of activity	Points
Golf (no motorized carts)	18 holes	3
Hockey*	20 min	3
Rope skipping (continuous)	5 min	1½
Skating*	15 min	1
Skiing*	30 min	3
Tennis	1 set	1½
Volleyball*	15 min	1
Wrestling*	5 min	2

*Only the time that is spent actively is to be counted.

ance, whereas sports such as golf, tennis, and volleyball produced very *minimal* contributions. The point values assigned to performance in several of these activities are presented in Table 12-2.

Laboratory experience

In the laboratory session or sessions devoted to explaining this program, each student should experience a number of different ways of earning an approximately equal number of points. In this way, the relative strenuousness of the activities can be compared by each individual. Also each person is introduced to different activities that can be used as part of this program. The instructor and the students may wish to select any number of the activities suggested in Table 12-3. The facilities available may dictate the activities that can be covered during the laboratory period. This work will be more meaningful if three or four different activities are used during the session. For additional activities, the reader is referred to the tables contained in *The New Aerobics*.

Most individuals find participating in activities such as tennis, golf, badminton, skiing, and skating more enjoyable than running, jumping rope continuously, or running in place for extended periods of time. If this is the case, it seems important for an individual to develop a skill level in at least one physical activity that could be used later in life, particularly when the student leaves college. Ideally, this activity should involve only one or two persons, and the more vigorous the activity is, the more beneficial it will be. Also, the skill level that is developed is a very important consideration. One's own skill level and that of the opponent determines to a large extent the vigorousness of the activity and the rate of energy expenditure.

CIRCUIT TRAINING

Circuit training is a form of general fitness training that evolved out of a search for a method that would both appeal to the students and also measurably increase their physical fitness level. It is based on sound physiological principles and was developed at the University of Leeds in 1955.[8]

Table 12-3. Suggested activities to be used for comparative purposes

Activity	Duration	Points
Rope skipping (continuous)	5 min	1½
Volleyball	23 min	1½
Basketball	10 min	1½
Stationary running	5 min (must complete approximately 350 steps*)	1½
Running/walking	1 mile in 12 min	2

*Count only when the left foot hits the floor.

The term *circuit* refers to a given number of exercises arranged and numbered consecutively in a given area. Each numbered exercise within the circuit is referred to as a *station*. The type of circuit that is set up is dependent on the time, space, and facilities available and the objectives desired for the program. The stations are usually located at approximately equal distances from each other and are designated by signs on the walls or bleachers that might surround the given area where the circuit is set up. These signs indicate the sequence for the activities and also the prescribed number of repetitions at each station.

The activities included in the circuit can be selected to achieve almost any objective in an attempt to develop the physical fitness components or the motor ability components or a combination of both. Also a circuit that is directed entirely to the development of specific skills can be set up.

Objectives

In circuit training each subject progresses at his own rate from one station to the next, performing a prescribed amount of work at each, until the entire circuit has been completed. Usually the single circuit is repeated several times, and the time for the total performance is recorded. The participants proceed from station to station without resting as they attempt to reduce the time taken for a given number of laps around the circuit. The basic assumption underlying circuit training is that improvement takes place either by doing the same amount of work in a shorter period of time or by doing more work in a given period of time. A student can progress by decreasing the time required to complete a given number of laps of the circuit or by increasing the number of repetitions performed at each station or by a combination of both of these methods.

The principle of progressive overload is stressed with circuit training. This principle is explained simply by Steinhaus:

> No matter how much a muscle is used, it will not grow larger or stronger until it is overloaded. This means that the intensity of the work required of it must be increased above that to which it is currently accustomed, i.e. it must be required to exert more power or work against a greater resistance than before.[12]

With circuit training, a progressive overload is built into the program by increasing the amount of work, increasing the rate of work, or decreasing the time factor.

Advantages

The basic advantage over other methods or calisthenics or programs of exercise is that circuit training stresses *continuous activity*. It has already been shown that continuous activity is a prerequisite for the development of the cardiovascular system. Unfortunately many of the exercise programs available today stress only muscular endurance and flexibility and place little emphasis on the development of cardiovascular endurance. Sorani[11] indicates that many students perform exercises of one type or another and that these exercises, if performed regularly and properly, can be worthwhile and satisfying. However, he indicates that frequently such exercise programs are not well planned or organized and that little thought is given to their purpose or procedure. Also many students participate in such exercise programs only when they like. When exercise is not performed on a regular basis, it is very difficult to include progressive overloading because lack of activity on a regular basis may result in regression. With circuit training, however, progression is built into the program, and each student should be working at his present capacity, since he progresses at his own rate. Circuit training, however, is no different from any other form of training in that the results depend entirely on the effort put forth by each participant.

Following is a list of the advantages associated with circuit training:

1. Each participant is able to commence this program at an easy pace and to experience some degree of success early in the program.
2. Circuit training can be organized so as to involve a large number of students in a relatively confined area.
3. Added motivation is provided by the fact that each participant can see his progress from day to day.
4. Progression is assured if the participant exercises regularly.
5. With circuit training the exercise is continuous, and thus stress is placed on the cardiovascular system.
6. Circuit training provides for individualized self-competition. Each participant is competing only against himself, and he works at his own individual rate.

Organization

Circuit training may be organized in a variety of different ways. Following is an example of the organization of a circuit consisting of eleven stations

Table 12-4. Circuit training activities

	I Yellow	II Black	III Red	IV Blue
1. Lateral jump	25	30	35	50
2. Hip raiser	10	12	16	25
3. Bent-leg sit-ups	10	15	20	30
4. Rope jump	40	50	60	80
5. Lateral leg raise	8	10	20	30
6. Burpee	8	10	20	30
7. Alternate toe-touch	20	25	35	40
8. V-sits	10	14	18	24
9. Push-ups	8	12	20	30
10. Bench jump	10	16	20	26
11. Sprinter	20	30	40	50

designed to develop the overall physical fitness of freshmen at the university level. This circuit is applicable for men and women students. A list of the activities and the repetitions for each of these are presented in Table 12-4.

Four progression levels have been established, although more may be added if they are needed. The initial starting level for each person can be determined by his performance on the 12-minute run test. Table 12-5 presents the criteria to be used in the determination of the starting level for each student. If the student has not taken this test, starting him at the lowest level and letting him progress from there is probably best.

Description of activities included in the circuit*

Lateral jump. Each subject jumps laterally across any line on the floor as fast as possible, keeping both feet together and parallel to the line. This activity develops muscular endurance of the legs as well as overall cardiovascular endurance.

*Several of these exercises are adapted from or similar to those suggested by Robert Sorani in his book *Circuit Training,* Dubuque, Iowa, 1966, Wm. C. Brown Co., pp. 45-62.

Table 12-5. Criteria for determination of the initial starting level for circuit training

Classification for 12-minute run test	Distance covered (miles)		Initial circuit level
	Men	Women	
Very poor or poor	Less than 1.24	Less than 1.19	Level I—Yellow circuit
Average	1.25-1.53	1.20-1.27	Level II—Black circuit
Good	1.57-1.84	1.28-1.42	Level III—Red circuit
Excellent	More than 1.84	More than 1.43	Level IV—Blue circuit

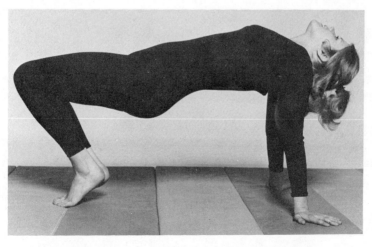

Fig. 12-1. Starting position for the hip raiser exercise.

Hip raiser. Each subject assumes the starting position as shown in Fig. 12-1. The hips are elevated as high as possible and then lowered as low as possible without the buttocks' touching the floor. This exercise will develop the muscular endurance of certain hip and thigh muscles as well as the abdominal muscles. It can be a good exercise to correct drooping shoulders.

Bent-leg sit-ups. This exercise is designed to strengthen the abdominal muscles and to increase their endurance. Each subject lies on his back on the floor with knees flexed at approximately 90° and feet placed flat on the floor. Flexing the knees places more stress on the abdominal muscles, and the muscles that flex the hip contribute less to the exercise. The fingers are interlocked and placed behind the neck (Fig. 7-1). The subject sits up so that at least one elbow touches one knee each time and then returns to the starting position. Each time he returns to the starting position, the fingers at the back of the head must come in contact with the floor.

Rope jump. This activity is designed for the development of cardiovascular endurance. A regular jump rope is used, and each subject must propel the rope in a counterclockwise direction so that it passes under his feet and over his head. Each time the rope passes under the feet counts as one repetition.

Lateral leg raise. Each subject assumes a position on the floor lying on either side with legs and lower arm completely extended and using the other arm to maintain his balance (Fig. 12-2). The upper leg is raised as high as possible, being kept straight, and is then returned slowly to the starting position. This constitutes one repetition. This exercise is designed to develop the muscles responsible for abduction of the leg. If the circuit is completed more than one time, the sides should be reversed, so that the leg that is raised is changed each time around the circuit.

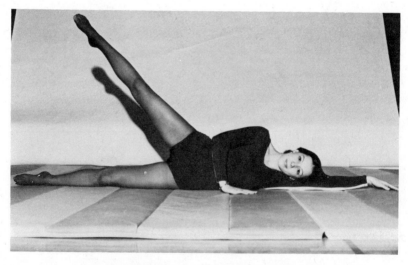

Fig. 12-2. Lateral leg raise exercise.

Burpee. This exercise is also referred to as the squat-thrust or the agility 4-count exercise. Each subject starts in a standing position with the legs straight. He assumes the squat position, extends the legs backward so that he assumes the push-up position, then reverses this procedure back to the squat position and finally back to the upright position. This completes one repetition. Because this exercise involves many large muscle groups, it contributes to over-all muscular endurance.

Alternate toe-touch. This exercise is a flexibility exercise designed to increase trunk flexion. Again the subject assumes an upright standing position with legs straight and feet shoulder-width apart. The arms are extended above the head. Keeping the legs straight, he reaches down to touch the left foot with the right hand, then returns to the starting position before reaching down again to touch the right foot with the left hand. When he returns again to the starting position, he has completed one repetition.

V-sits. The subject lies on the floor on his back at the start of this activity with arms extended fully behind the head. He then curls the head toward the chest as the arms and legs are raised simultaneously until a V-position is obtained (Fig. 12-3). The subject then reverses these procedures until the starting position is reached. This exercise is a good one for the development of the abdominal muscles, particularly if the V-position is maintained for a few seconds each time.

Push-ups. Men should perform the regular push-up, starting from the front-leaning rest position with the head, back, hips, and legs in a straight

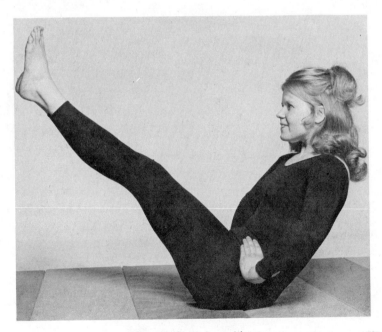

Fig. 12-3. V-sit position.

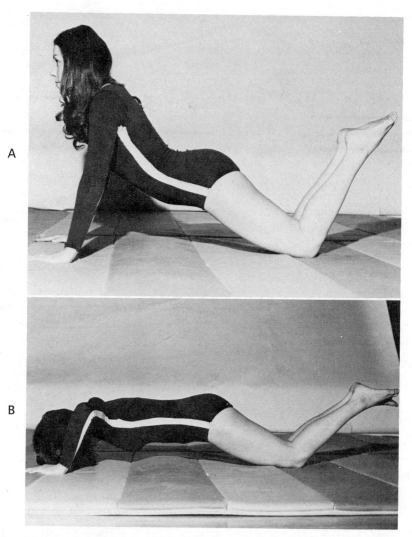

Fig. 12-4. Starting **(A)** and finishing **(B)** positions for the modified push-up for women.

alignment. The body is slowly lowered so that the chest lightly touches the floor. The body should remain straight throughout this exercise. The arms are then extended, as the body is raised to the starting position. This exercise will develop the muscular endurance and strength of the extensors of the forearm. Women should perform the modified push-up (Fig. 12-4) or the alternate method for the push-up, using the lowest row of bleachers for support (Fig. 12-5).

Bench jump or bench step. For this activity the subject faces a bench that is approximately 12 to 16 inches high. The lowest row of bleachers is

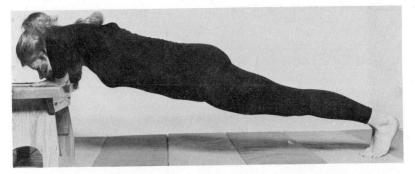

Fig. 12-5. Alternate method of push-ups for women.

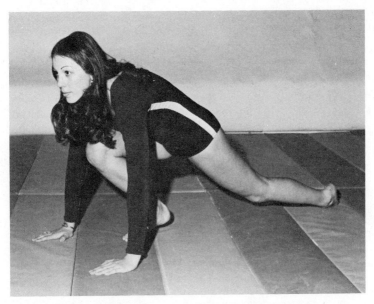

Fig. 12-6. Position to be assumed for the sprinter exercise.

usually satisfactory for this exercise. The subject jumps up onto and down from the bench. This completes one repetition. If he is unable to jump onto the bench, he should step up, following the same procedure that is used for the step test. This exercise is designed to develop cardiovascular endurance as well as strength and endurance of the leg extensors.

Sprinter. The subject assumes a position similar to a sprinter's starting position, with the weight on the hands and feet with one leg extended straight back and the other flexed with the knee pulled under the chest (Fig. 12-6). The position of the feet is then reversed and reversed again as the subject returns to the starting position. This completes one repetition. This exercise contributes to the development of strength and endurance of the shoulder and arm extensors as well as leg flexors and extensors.

Instructions for running a circuit

All students should be provided with the following information before the circuit is attempted. In addition, each exercise should be demonstrated to the students, and they should each have a chance to practice the exercise so that it may be performed correctly.

1. Fifteen minutes will be allowed for each male and 18 minutes for each female student to complete two laps of the circuit.
2. If the two laps around the circuit are completed before the allocated time has elapsed, the remainder of the time is to be spent completing as many single laps across the badminton court as are possible in the remaining time. The same procedures that apply to the 3-minute shuttle run will apply here. These procedures are outlined in Chapter 5.
3. If a subject completes twenty or more laps within the time limit, the next time he attempts the circuit, he should move up to the next level.
4. A person who fails to complete two entire laps of the circuit in the prescribed time and is not working at level I should move back one level the next time that he attempts the circuit.
5. To measure progress each day each student should record the total time taken to complete two laps of the circuit and also the number of laps across the badminton court completed within the prescribed time limit.

WALKING-JOGGING-RUNNING PROGRAM

Running as a method for the development of physical fitness is looked upon unfavorably by many people. However "such an image of running only reflects a poor understanding of this versatile means of activity. Running as a means of obtaining a feeling of well-being need not, and should not, be an unpleasant experience nor should it be a daily challenge of man's ability to survive physical adversity."*

Definition of terms

Certain terms must be defined for a clear understanding of the following material that is presented in this unit:

walking Form of movement in which at least one foot is in contact with the ground at all times.

jogging Form of running, at a slow to moderate pace. Balke clarifies this definition by stating that "jogging is running at a speed which can be equalled or surpassed by fast walking."

running Form of movement during which no more than one foot may be in contact with the ground at any one time or both feet are off the ground during a portion of each stride.

---

*From Balke, B.: Guidelines for walking-jogging-running training mimeographed material, Madison, University of Wisconsin, p. 1. Portions of this discussion are summarized from this material.

interval running Intermittent running in which a given distance is repeated several times with a rest interval between each run. The "rest" may be in the form of walking, jogging, or complete rest.

Brisk walking, jogging, or running may be used for a variety of reasons. Probably the fundamental purpose is to increase one's cardiovascular endurance. By progressively making the task more difficult, the development of the circulatory system takes place, and the body is capable of using more oxygen.[4]

Secondary objectives as presented by Roby and Davis[9] include "the improvement of appearance through weight or figure control and better posture, together with improvement of those psychological traits which have to do with inner confidence, will-power and the ability to resist both mental and physical stress."

Variation of the program

The strenuousness of the program can be varied by any one of the following: (1) regulating the distance covered, (2) adjusting the ratio of walking to running, or (3) adjusting the speed of running. The program needs to be adapted to the age and fitness levels of the participants as realistic objectives are established.

Advantages of a jogging program*

Following is a list of advantages associated with a well-designed jogging or running program:

1. Simple and most effective way to stimulate the circulation and exercise the heart
2. Superior to many other forms of exercise in that it provides a gentle, steady, and prolonged demand on the heart rather than a series of short but severe ones
3. Provides for the development of body flexibility and exercises most parts of the body
4. Can be adapted to the physical fitness and age level of each participant
5. Can be performed at any time and place
6. Requires no special equipment or facilities, and the costs involved are very minimal
7. Takes little time
8. Requires little learning skill, since it is a natural activity

Development of a jogging program

In designing a jogging or running program the following guidelines may be helpful:[10]

1. Begin by walking daily, increasing the speed of walking until you can walk briskly for 10 minutes without overexertion.

---

*The material in this section is summarized from *Running Into Fitness,* a pamphlet produced by the National Fitness Council of South Australia.

2. Next, alternate jogging with walking for a total of 10 minutes daily. Gradually increase the amount of jogging as you spend less time walking until you are able to jog continuously for 10 minutes.
3. Finally, increase the length of time spent jogging daily and also increase the speed of jogging as your endurance increases. You will progress from jogging to running.
4. You need to run at least every second day. If you can make this 5 or 6 days per week, the training effects should occur much more quickly.
5. It is not important to concentrate on running style, but beginners should try placing the ball and heel of the foot first and not the toes. Relaxation of the ankles, knees, hips, shoulders, face, and hands should also be considered. The more relaxed the person is, the easier it is for him to run.

For further details concerning standardized jogging and running programs that have been developed for persons of all ages, see the program suggested by Bowerman and Harris[1] or the program by Roby and Davis.[9]

Changes that take place as a result of jogging and running

A report by Wilmore[13] indicates that jogging is an excellent form of exercise, provided that a medical examination is obtained before the beginning of the program, the program is started gradually, and each participant avoids competing with his friends. He indicated that as a result of an 11-week jogging program, the following changes resulted: (1) an 8% decrease in body fat, (2) a significant increase in vital capacity, (3) a 10% to 13% decrease in resting blood pressure, (4) a 12% decrease in the resting heart rate, and (5) a significant decrease in the cholesterol and triglyceride levels.

INTERVAL TRAINING

Not all exercise programs need to be performed continuously. For example, in an exercise program designed to lose weight, the total amount of work performed is most important. The more work that is performed, the more Calories are used, and thus the greater the loss in weight. Whether this work is performed continuously is not important. It has been shown clearly that when a task is broken up into bouts of short duration with intervening periods of rest, greater total work loads can be performed. This type of training is referred to as interval training.[2] Actually, there are four variables involved with interval training, any one or all of which can be altered to change the intensity of the task—(1) the distance to be run, (2) the amount of time taken to run this distance, (3) the number of times this distance to be run (repetitions), and (4) the amount of time allowed for rest between each run. An example should help to make this information more meaningful. Interval training for a specific situation might involve running four repetitions of 100 yards each, at full speed, with a 20-second rest interval between each bout. Any one or all of the four variables could be altered to change the intensity of the task. A much more strenuous task might be running eight repetitions of

220 yards each in 45 seconds with a 2-minute rest interval between each repetition. With this task, if a participant takes less than 45 seconds to run the 220 yards, he has the additional time added to his rest period. A person who takes longer than 45 seconds to run the 220 yards would actually have less than a 2-minute rest between repetitions.

Laboratory experience

The laboratory work that each person can experience with this unit will vary according to the facilities available. Following are several suggestions that might be included:

1. Each student should jog continuously at a comfortable pace for a 10-minute period. The pace will be determined by each student, and at the completion of the jog he should feel comfortable and not be exhausted. Each subject should calculate the distance covered, and the point table (Table 12-1) should be consulted to determine how many points this would earn in the aerobics program. It should be stressed that the aim of this is *not* to cover the greatest possible distance but merely to establish a comfortable jogging speed for a 10-minute period of time.

Distance covered in 10 minutes
at a moderate jogging speed = _____ miles

Speed = _____ miles × 6

= _____ miles/hr

2. Each student can be introduced to an interval training program designed to develop speed and power. Each student should select at least one of the following tasks.[6]

   a. Ten repetitions of 100 yards each in 18 seconds with 110-yard walk interval between each run

   b. Twenty repetitions of 60 yards each in 9 seconds with a 30-second rest interval between each run

   c. Thirty repetitions of 40 yards each in 6 seconds with a 20-second rest interval between each run

3. Each student can participate in an interval-training program designed to develop cardiovascular endurance. Again each instructor or class should select at least one of the following tasks:[4]

   a. Three repetitions of 880 yards each in 3½ minutes with a 5-minute rest interval between each run

   b. Six repetitions of 440 yards each in 100 seconds with a 2-minute rest interval between each run

   c. Two repetitions of 1 mile each in 9 minutes with a 3-minute rest interval between each run

Summary

There are many different methods available to vary the walking-jogging-running program. By varying the program from day to day, each person is much more likely to maintain his initial motivation. Remember that walking, jogging, and running can be a lot of fun.

EXERCISE PROGRAM FOR ALLEVIATION OF LOW BACK PAIN

That the great majority of persons who suffer from low back pain can alleviate the problem by regular exercise has been clearly demonstrated. However, the choice of exercises is very important. Ones that will strengthen the abdominal musculature and lengthen the hamstring muscle group must be selected. Kraus[6] has shown that the following exercises are most beneficial as far as the elimination of low back pain is concerned.

1. *Bent-knee sit-ups.* Instructions are the same as those for item 2 of the Kraus-Weber test.
2. *Toe touches.* The instructions for this activity are the same as those for item 6 of the Kraus-Weber test.
3. *Back hyperextension.* The subject assumes a prone position with a pillow under his pelvis. With feet held and arms straight and at his side, the upper body is lifted off the floor until the legs and body are in a straight line.
4. *Back arch.* The subject assumes a kneeling position on "all fours" on the floor. The back is arched upward as far as possible from the floor. In this position the head should be lowered so that the forehead is as close to the floor as possible. Next, the back is "dropped" to a swayback position, and the head is lifted so that the forehead is as far away from the floor as possible.
5. *Leg curls.* The subject assumes a supine position on the floor. With hands behind the neck, the legs are slowly lifted, the knees are bent, and the legs are curled until the knees are in contact with the chest. The legs are then straightened and lowered to the starting position.

Other exercise programs are available for alleviation of low back pain and for building a stronger back. Feffer suggests that the following eight exercises be performed twice a day, starting with four repetitions and increasing to ten. The exercises he recommends are as follows:

Lying on stomach

1. Pinch buttocks together. Pull stomach in. Hold position for five seconds, then relax five seconds. Over a period of days, increase holding-relaxing period to 20 seconds.

Lying on back

2. Bend knees with feet flat on floor, keeping arms at sides. Pinch buttocks together. Pull in stomach and flatten lower back against floor. Hold for five seconds, relax for five seconds. Gradually build up to 20 seconds.
3. Repeat exercise 2 with legs extended.
4. Draw knees toward chest. Clasp hands around knees. Keep shoulders flat against floor. Pull knees tightly against chest, then bring forehead to knees.

5. Bend knees with feet flat on floor; cross arms on chest. Raise head and shoulders from floor. Curl up to sitting position. Keep back round and pull with stomach muscles. Lower self slowly.

6. Bend knees, keeping feet flat on floor and arms straight forward. Touch head to knees. Lower self. Draw knees toward chest. Pull knees tightly against chest and bring forehead to knees.

Sitting on floor

7. Keep legs straight. Pull stomach in. Reach forward with hands and try to touch toes with fingers. Use rocking motion.

Sitting on a chair

8. Place hands at edge of chair. Bend forward to bring head to knees, pulling stomach in as you curl forward. Keep weight well back on hips. Release stomach muscles slowly as you come up.*

*Reprinted from U.S. News & World Report, Sept. 20, 1971. Copyright 1971 U.S. News & World Report, Inc.

REFERENCES

1. Bowerman, W. J., and Harris, W. E.: Jogging, New York, 1967, Grosset & Dunlap, Inc.
2. Cooper, K. H.: New aerobics, New York, 1972, Bantam Books, Inc.
3. De Vries, H. A.: Physiology of exercise for physical education and athletics, ed. 4, London, 1968, Staples Press, Ltd., pp. 219, 333-335.
4. Harris, W. E., and Bowerman, W.: Jogging—an adult exercise program, The Journal of the American Medical Association **201:**759, 1967.
5. Howell, M. L., and Morford, W. R.: Circuit training for a college fitness program, Journal of Health, Physical Education and Recreation **35:**30, 1964.
6. Kraus, H.: Backache, stress and tension; their cause, prevention and treatment, New York, 1965, Simon & Schuster, Inc.
7. Landers, D., and Wade, M.: The University of Illinois foundations laboratory handbook.
8. Morgan, R. E., and Adamson, G. T.: Circuit training, London, 1957, G. Bell & Sons, Ltd.
9. Roby, F. B., and Davis, R. P.: Jogging for fitness and weight control, Philadelphia, 1970, W. B. Saunders Company, pp. 1-109.
10. Run for your life program provokes a physician debate, Medical Tribune, Oct. 12, 1967.
11. Sorani, R.: Circuit training, Dubuque, Iowa, 1966, Wm. C. Brown Company, Publishers, pp. 45-62.
12. Steinhaus, A. H.: Strength from Mofungo to Mueller—a half century of research, Journal of the Association for Physical and Mental Rehabilitation **9:**147, Sept.-Oct., 1955.
13. Wilmore, J. H.: Benefits derived from an eleven week jogging program, Medicine in Sports, p. 4, Nov. 9, 1969.

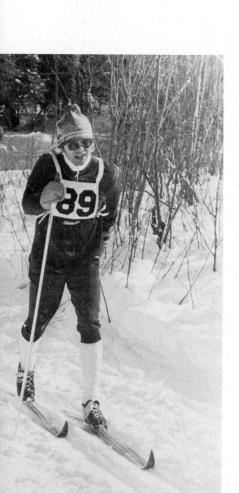

chapter 13

Relative value of various activities in the development of physical fitness

What do you know about the contribution of various activities to the development of physical fitness?

T   F

__ __ **1.** For an activity to contribute to the development of physical fitness it must produce a near maximal heart rate.

__ __ **2.** Maximal heart rate will not change drastically as one ages.

__ __ **3.** Activities that require continuous action and involve large muscle groups will generally be good for the development of cardiovascular endurance.

__ __ **4.** Tennis is a good activity for the development of cardiovascular endurance.

__ __ **5.** One of the best activities for the development of cardiovascular endurance is basketball.

__ __ **6.** An activity must produce a heart rate of 140 to 150 beats per minute and sustain this for 5 minutes to be beneficial for the development of cardiovascular endurance.

__ __ **7.** Football is a very poor activity for the development of cardiovascular fitness.

In designing an exercise program, it is important to know how strenuous an activity must be to contribute toward the development of cardiovascular fitness and which activities can best be used for this purpose.

CRITICAL HEART RATE

It has been shown that if an activity is to contribute to the development of cardiovascular fitness, there is a critical heart rate that must be exceeded. Working with untrained subjects, Karvonen[5] found that if an activity was to improve the exercise tolerance of the heart, it must produce a heart rate in excess of the value located 60% of the way between the resting and the maximal heart rates. For most of these subjects, this critical value was between 140 and 150 beats per minute. The resting heart rate may be determined very easily. This should be taken several times to make sure that the value is a typical value for the subject involved. The maximal heart rate can be estimated as follows:

Estimated maximal heart rate $= 220 -$ age (years)

$$= 220 - \underline{\hspace{3cm}}$$

$$= \underline{\hspace{4cm}}$$

Resting heart rate $= \underline{\hspace{4cm}}$ Trial 1

$$= \underline{\hspace{4cm}}$$ Trial 2

$$= \underline{\hspace{4cm}}$$ Trial 3

$$= \underline{\hspace{4cm}}$$ Trial 4

Typical score $= \underline{\hspace{4cm}}$ beats/minute

Evaluation of critical heart rate

Critical heart rate $=$ Resting heart rate $+ .60$ (Maximal heart rate $-$ Resting heart rate)

Example: If a subject has a resting heart rate of 70 beats per minute and a maximal heart rate of 190 beats per minute . . .

$$\begin{aligned}
\text{Critical heart rate} &= 70 + .60 \ (190 - 70) \\
&= 70 + .60 \ (120) \\
&= 70 + 72 \\
&= 142
\end{aligned}$$

Each person should calculate his own critical heart rate.

$$\text{Critical heart rate} = \underline{\hspace{1.5cm}} + .60 \ (\underline{\hspace{1.5cm}} - \underline{\hspace{1.5cm}})$$

$$= \underline{\hspace{1.5cm}} + .60 \ (\qquad)$$

$$= \underline{\hspace{1.5cm}} + \underline{\hspace{1.5cm}}$$

$$= \underline{\hspace{1.5cm}}$$

Cooper[2] has indicated that for maximal development of cardiovascular endurance an activity must produce a heart rate in excess of 150 beats per minute and that such improvement begins only after this rate of activity has been

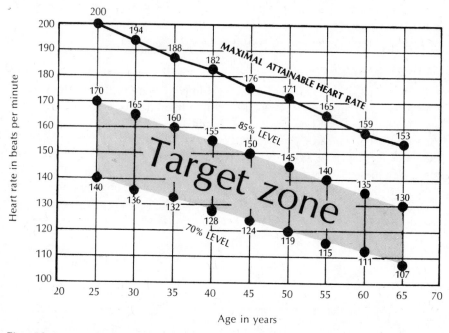

Fig. 13-1. Summary of changes that take place as a result of age as far as the maximal attainable heart rate is concerned and what the target zone is for each age group. The numerical values shown are "average" values for each age. (Courtesy Best Foods Division, CPC International, Englewood Cliffs, N.J.)

sustained for at least 5 minutes. In addition to this, the activity must be performed a minimum of three or four times per week.

The American Heart Association[8] suggests that there is a target zone as far as heart rate is concerned that is sufficient to develop cardiovascular fitness but not too high to exceed safe limits. They suggest that this target zone is between 60% and 85% of a person's maximal aerobic power. Below 60% of his capacity, a person achieves very little fitness benefit while above 85% there is very little added benefit. The maximal attainable heart rates and the target zones for different age groups are presented in Fig. 13-1.

RELATIVE STRENUOUSNESS OF VARIOUS ACTIVITIES

To learn which activities are most stressful to the heart and can be used when an overload is necessary for the development of cardiovascular endurance is important. Identifying activities that are less stressful also is important. This information allows the individual to increase the efficiency of his heart by overloading it at times and allowing it to slow down at other times.

In activities such as running, swimming, and bicycling the strenuousness will be determined by how fast one performs. This, of course, is related to how much time is taken to cover a specified distance. The reader is referred to tables in the Cooper book that have been based on these criteria.

DETERMINATION OF THE STRENUOUSNESS OF AN ACTIVITY

Without some form of telemetry equipment, it is difficult to determine the heart rate during participation in most activities. An alternate method is to determine the pulse immediately upon completing the exercise. It is important to count immediately because the rate changes very quickly once exercise is slowed or stopped. The American Heart Association recommends that you find the beat within one second of the end of exercise, count for 10 seconds, and multiply this by 6 to convert this to beats per minute. They suggest that this is superior to counting for the whole minute or for 15 seconds because the "drop-off" is too fast.

Several studies have been conducted comparing different activities. Balke[1] has conducted research comparing eleven different activities. In this study the maximum capacity is expressed in Mets. One Met is equivalent to the energy a person uses while sitting at rest. The eleven activities are listed in Table 13-1 in order of the maximal capacity in Mets.

The National Athletic Health Institute[6] has released figures comparing various groups of athletes. Their unit for comparative purposes is maximal oxygen uptake expressed in milliliters of oxygen per kilogram of body weight (ml/kg Bw). The maximal oxygen uptake of an individual represents the best estimate available for cardiovascular fitness and endurance capacity. The reason for this is that all living cells require oxygen to function properly, and as you increase your muscular activity the oxygen demanded by your muscles increases in direct proportion. There is a definite limit with regard to how much oxygen your body can supply. Theoretically, the higher this value, the higher the level of cardiovascular fitness.

Maximal oxygen uptake figures for twelve different sports are provided in Table 13-2.

Table 13-1. Maximal capacity in Mets of athletes[3]

Sport	Maximal capacity in Mets
Track running	23
Cross country skiing	23
Speed skating	23
Rowing	19
Cycling	18
Competitive swimming	18
Alpine skiing	16
Ice hockey	16
Basketball	15½
Tennis	13
Football	13

Table 13-2. Maximal oxygen uptake in milliliters per kilograms of body weight

Sport	Maximal O₂ uptake (average figures— ml O₂/kg Bw)
Cross country skiing	70-94
Long distance running	65-85
Rowing	58-75
Bicycling	55-70
Basketball	55-70
Speed skating	50-75
Ice hockey	50-60
Distance swimming	48-68
Gymnastics	48-64
Football	45-64
Baseball	45-55
Tennis	42-56

The results presented in Table 13-2 show that the five sports that rank highest all require continuous sustained action over a long period of time and involve the use of large muscle groups.

The sports that ranked near the bottom of the list, such as football, baseball and tennis, do not involve continuous activity. In tennis it was found that over 50% of the time was spent standing around getting ready to play and *not* in actual competition.

A similar comparison was conducted by Golding[7] of Kent State University. He compared ten different sports and ranked them according to the level of cardiovascular fitness of participants. His rankings were as follows: (1) track, (2) swimming, (3) cross-country, (4) soccer, (5) ice hockey, (6) basketball, (7) football, (8) tennis, (9) baseball, and (10) golf.

Several studies have shown that neither golf nor weight lifting produce a heart rate in excess of the threshold value required to produce a training effect. Weight lifters, despite their well-developed skeletal system, rate no higher than the average untrained subject as far as cardiovascular endurance is concerned. Getchell[4] studied the effect of a season of golf for twenty middle-aged golfers who averaged over 12 hours per week on the golf course. When compared to the sedentary control group of subjects, there was very little difference on their response to a submaximal work task.

It appears as if activities can be classified into four groups according to the contributions they might make toward the development of cardiovascular fitness. These arbitary classifications are as follows:

Group 1. Low contribution
  Archery Calisthenics
  Bowling Golf
  Baseball Volleyball

Group 2. Minimal contribution
  Gymnastics
  Tennis
  Football

Group 3. High contribution

Badminton
Basketball
Rowing
Judo
Snowshoeing

Group 4. Very high contribution

Bicycling	Soccer
Handball	Swimming
Paddleball	Cross-country skiing
Squash	Wrestling
Running	

SUMMARY

Various studies clearly indicate that activities involving continuous activity and large muscle groups can be used to develop cardiovascular endurance. Activities that result in a heart rate in excess of 140 to 150 beats per minute and that is continued at this rate for extended periods of time appear to be most beneficial. Research indicates that activities such as running, cross-country skiing, skating, rowing, bicycling, swimming, hiking, handball, paddleball, basketball, and orienteering are some of the activities that rate high. Activities such as weight lifting, football, volleyball, golf, and calisthenics rate low when evaluated according to these criteria.

REFERENCES

1. Balke, B.: Rank of apparent benefits of various activities in Mets, Proceedings of American College of Sports Medicine, May, 1971.
2. Cooper, K., and Brown, K.: Aerobics, New York, 1968, M. Evans and Company, Inc.
3. Cundiff, D. E.: Fundamentals of functional fitness, Dubuque, Iowa, 1974, Kendall/ Hunt Publishing Company, p. 67.
4. Getchell, L. H., Energy cost of playing golf, Archives of Physical Medicine 49:31-35, Jan., 1968.
5. Karvonen, M. J.: Effects of vigorous exercise on the heart. In Rosenbaum, F. F., and Belknap, E. L., editors: Work and the heart, New York, 1959, Paul B. Hoeber, Inc.
6. National Athletic Health Institute, printed information, California, 1975.
7. President's Council on Physical Fitness and Sports: Newsletter, Washington, D.C., Aug.-Sept., 1973, p. 4.
8. Zohman, L. R.: Exercise your way to fitness and heart health, American Heart Association, 1974, p. 11.

chapter 14
Developing an exercise program

___ ___ **1.** Exercising for one hour per week is as beneficial as exercising for ten minutes daily.

___ ___ **2.** Progressive resistance is no longer necessary once a desired level of fitness has been reached.

___ ___ **3.** Overload is a form of physical stress.

___ ___ **4.** Intensity and duration of physical exercises provide the primary means by which activity may become progressively more strenuous.

___ ___ **5.** An overload is any exercise that exceeds in intensity or duration the demands usually made on the organism.

___ ___ **6.** Most existing exercise programs are good for the development of cardiovascular fitness.

___ ___ **7.** A person must exercise every day if he wants to improve his level of physical fitness.

___ ___ **8.** A person need only exercise 10 minutes per day to bring about maximal development of physical fitness.

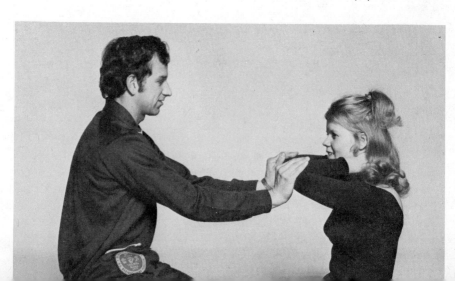

The preceding chapters have presented information relative to the importance of regular physical activity. The reasons for maintaining a desirable level of physical fitness and body weight have been discussed. Along with this information, a series of tests were also presented so that each individual could carefully evaluate his present level of fitness, motor ability, and nutritional status. Several different exercise programs have been summarized that can be used for improving one's level of fitness.

All this information has been presented in the hope that persons may realize just how unfit they really are and may do something about it. Having knowledge concerning physical fitness is not sufficient; the knowledge must be applied and used. Each person must believe strongly enough in the importance of physical fitness to do something about it. Knowing and talking about it are not sufficient.

PRINCIPLES OF EXERCISE

There are certain basic principles that need to be followed if a good exercise program is to result.

1. *It takes time and effort to develop an adequate level of physical fitness.* No "short-cut," easy methods exist. Dr. Cureton states that "the first thing you must do is to face the fact that there are no short cuts. It will take three months of hard work—possibly the hardest work of your life—before you see significant changes."[1] For this reason the development of physical fitness should be a lifetime matter. Ideally, an adequate level of physical fitness should be developed early and be maintained throughout life.[3] It has been suggested that physical fitness should be considered as existing on a continuum or scale (Fig. 4-2). The amount and type of physical activity that each person includes in his daily routine will determine to a large extent his position on this scale. If exercise is not continued throughout life, there will be a decrease in the level of physical fitness.

2. *The program should be designed to meet the present needs of the individual.* Much time and energy can be wasted unless certain specific goals are established for a program. These goals should be based on the needs of each individual. It has been emphasized that the level of physical fitness necessary will vary. Some persons need a much higher level of physical fitness than others.

After an individual has established his specific goals, he must be able to evaluate carefully his progress as he strives to attain his objectives. There is no exercise program that is good for everyone. Each has to be designed to suit the needs, abilities, and goals of each person.

3. *A well-planned program will be directed toward the improvement of each component of physical fitness.* It has been emphasized that physical fitness involves strength, flexibility, and muscular and cardiovascular endurance. A good exercise program must be directed toward the development of all four components. It has also been stressed that of these four components cardiovascular endurance is the most important health benefit. Therefore the de-

velopment of this component should occupy a prominent position in any exercise program.

4. *The program must be systematic.* All too frequently exercise is performed irregularly, with little thought given to the reasons for specific exercises. Exercises must be organized into a systematic program designed to meet the basic needs of each individual.

5. *Regular participation in any exercise program is necessary.* To achieve specific objectives, participation must be on a regular basis. Persons who wait until they "find" time to exercise do not exercise very often. If they believe strongly enough in the importance of exercise, they will make time available on a regular basis. Exercise should become a habit, and if possible, it should be scheduled at a regular time each day. An exercise program can be considered regular when participation occurs at least four times a week.

6. *An overload is the key to a successful program.* For significant improvement to take place, an overload is necessary—meaning simply that it is necessary to subject the body to a task slightly beyond its normal level. DeVries indicates that "whether we are concerned with strength, muscular endurance, or cardiovascular endurance, improvement in function occurs only when the system involved is challenged. Improvement occurs when, and only when, the workload is greater than that to which the individual is accustomed."[2] It should be stressed that overload is not the same as overwork. Overloading involves placing enough stress on the body to stimulate the desired response without resulting in exhaustion.

7. *Progression is an important part of every exercise program.* The body will adapt to an increased level of resistance as improvement takes place. For this reason it is necessary to measure progress and to increase the work load frequently. It should also be emphasized that it is not wise to commence a vigorous program if one is accustomed to a sedentary way of life. The program should be moderate at first, and then progression will be incorporated as the body is able to adapt to the increased stress level. Students should not be discouraged by lack of progress at different times during the program. Progress is quickest and most apparent at the start of a program, particularly if the person has been inactive prior to the start of the program. Progress slows down as one approaches his maximal potential, since the more he progresses, the harder it is to keep improving. It is only through increasing the workload that progression will be possible.

8. *A training program will result in specificity of improvement.* An exercise program is specific and will result in improvement only in the area or areas that it is designed to develop. For example, a person who lifts weights regularly will develop strength and muscular endurance only. Similarly, unless a person includes activities that involve large muscle groups and that result in heart rates that exceed 150 beats per minute for extended periods of time, he should not expect to experience a notable improvement in cardiovascular endurance. The activities that make up the program will determine the results attained. The system adapts to the specific exercise attempted. A person who engages

in walking becomes fit for walking, while a person who trains on a bicycle becomes a better bicyclist. A person who runs gets in shape for running. There is little carry-over from one activity to another.

FREQUENCY OF THE EXERCISE PROGRAM

Research indicates that a good exercise program should be performed at least four times per week and possibly not more than five times per week. Rest periods are essential and should be built into any exercise program. They result in both physical and mental relaxation.

LENGTH OF EACH EXERCISE SESSION

The length of each exercise session may vary according to the specific objectives. It appears that the proposed plan as recommended by the American Heart Association is adequate for most people. They suggest that each exercise session be divided into three segments as follows:

1. A 5- to 10-minute warm-up session so that the heart and circulatory system are not suddenly taxed
2. A sustained 20- to 30-minute exercise series in which the heart rate remains in the target zone
3. A 5- to 10-minute cool-down session in which the intensity of the task is, lessened before exercise is stopped

This plan is summarized in Fig. 14-1.

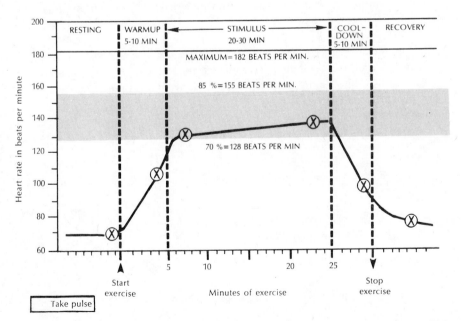

Fig. 14-1. Suggested exercise training pattern. (Courtesy Best Foods Division, CPC International, Englewood Cliffs, N.J.)

SELECTION OF ACTIVITIES

The reader is referred to Chapter 13 to determine which activities might be best for increasing the heart rate to the desired level. This will also depend upon the skill of the exerciser, the fitness level of the exerciser, the pattern of rest pauses, and the environmental temperature. It is suggested that each person vary his program so as to maintain interest and motivation.

No matter which activities are selected, each person should check his heart rate as indicated above to make sure that the intensity is adequate to raise the heart rate to the desired level.

SEMESTER ASSIGNMENT

The laboratory assignment for the semester might include the development of a 3-month personal physical fitness program based on the individual needs of each student. The assignment should include the following:

1. A summary concerning the student's present physical fitness level. Each student should make use of the results of the tests that relate to physical fitness. These should be presented in a meaningful way with a conclusion concerning the student's present physical fitness level.

2. A statement concerning the objectives or goals that each student establishes for his physical fitness program. These should be presented in terms of pupil behavior and should state specifically what each student will be able to demonstrate if he successfully completes his program and attains the desired results.

3. Information relating to the activities included in the program. This section should include the following:

a. A list of activities.

b. The specific purposes for each activity proposed.

c. Samples of weekly schedules showing the amount of each exercise or activity. They should also demonstrate how progression is built into the program.

d. Procedures to be followed for evaluation of progress toward the desired goals.

REFERENCES

1. Cureton, T. K.: Run for your life. In The healthy life, New York, 1966, Time, Inc., p. 36.
2. DeVries, H. A.: Physiology of exercise for physical education and athletics, Dubuque, Iowa, 1966, Wm. C. Brown Company, Publishers, p. 218.
3. Hanson, D.: Health related fitness, Belmont, Calif., 1970, Wadsworth Publishing Co., Inc., p. 4.

ACTIVITY INVENTORY*

Now that you have completed this course, it is important to find out which activities you are actively engaged in and which ones you would like to learn more about.

Place a check mark in column 1 next to each activity that you have participated in regularly for at least 8 weeks any time during the last 12 months.

Place a check mark in column 2 next to each activity that you would like to learn more about and in which you would like to increase your skill level.

Numbers are included next to each activity so that computer cards may be used for tabulating results where desired. Students will use the number corresponding to each activity and make their responses next to that number on the IBM card.

INDIVIDUAL AND DUAL SPORTS

	Col. 1	Col. 2
1. Archery		
2. Badminton		
3. Bowling		
4. Calisthenics		
5. Fencing		
6. Fly casting		
7. Golf		
8. Gymnastics		
9. Handball		
10. Hiking		
11. Jogging		
12. Judo		
13. Paddle ball		
14. Skating		
15. Skiing		
16. Tennis		
17. Track and field		
18. Weight lifting		
19. Wrestling		

DANCE

	Col. 1	Col. 2
20. Ballet		
21. Ballroom		
22. Creative		
23. Folk		
24. Square		

TEAM SPORTS

	Col. 1	Col. 2
25. Baseball		
26. Basketball		
27. Field hockey		
28. Ice hockey		
29. Softball		
30. Soccer		
31. Touch football		
32. Volleyball		

AQUATICS

	Col. 1	Col. 2
33. Canoeing		
34. Diving		
35. Lifesaving		
36. Sailing		
37. Swimming		
38. Water safety instruction (WSI)		

OTHERS (LIST)

	Col. 1	Col. 2

*Adapted from Humphrey, J. H., and Ingram, A. G.: Introduction to physical education for college students, Boston, 1969, Holbrook Press, p. 37.

ATTITUDE QUESTIONNAIRE

Now that you have completed this course, it is important to see what effect this class has had on your attitude toward exercise and physical education. Please respond to each of the following questions by placing a check mark in the appropriate column. Again you are asked to be honest and objective in your answers.

Age _____ Sex _____

Laboratory instructor _____

	Strongly agree	Agree	Undecided	Disagree	Strongly disagree
1. Little learning takes place in physical education classes.					
2. At the college level, physical education classes contribute little and do not justify the time and money spent on them.					
3. Physical education classes should be offered at the college level, but whether they take them or not ought to be up to the students.					
4. Most information about exercises and physical fitness is common knowledge.					
5. Physical education should consist only of those activities that are fun to participate in.					
6. I would take physical education classes only if they were a university requirement.					
7. Physical education should develop in students an understanding of the importance of exercise to health and fitness.					
8. All required subjects at the college level in all areas should be offered only as electives, except for the area that the student is majoring in.					
9. Most adults get all the exercise they need by performing their daily tasks.					
10. The development of an adequate level of physical fitness should be a worthwhile objective for all college students.					
11. This class contained little information of interest to me and was definitely a waste of time.					
12. All students at the college level should be exposed to such a course as this.					
13. I am now more active during my leisure hours than I was before I took this class.					

Index